Staff Nurse Survival Guide

Staff Nurse Survival Guide
2nd Edition

Edited by

John Fowler

QUAY
BOOKS

A division of MA Healthcare Ltd

John Fowler is series editor for the following titles:

Fundamental Aspects of Adult Nursing Procedures
Fundamental Aspects of Caring for the Person with Dementia
Fundamental Aspects of Children and Young People's Nursing Procedures
Fundamental Aspects of Community Nursing
Fundamental Aspects of Complementary Therapies
Fundamental Aspects of Finding Information
Fundamental Aspects of Gynaecology Nursing
Fundamental Aspects of Legal, Ethical and Professional Issues in Nursing
Fundamental Aspects of Men's Health
Fundamental Aspects of Mental Health Nursing
Fundamental Aspects of Nursing the Acutely Ill Adult
Fundamental Aspects of Nursing Adults with Respiratory Disorders
Fundamental Aspects of Pain Assessment and Management
Fundamental Aspects of Palliative Care Nursing (2nd Edition)
Fundamental Aspects of Tissue Viability
Fundamental Aspects of Transcultural Nursing
Fundamental Aspects of Women's Health

Quay Books Division, MA Healthcare Ltd, St Jude's Church, Dulwich Road,
London SE24 0PB

British Library Cataloguing-in-Publication Data
A catalogue record is available for this book

© MA Healthcare Limited 2010
ISBN 10: 1-85642-397-2
ISBN 13: 978-1-85642-397-7

Printed in the UK by CLE Huntingdon, Cambridgeshire

Contents

Introduction to the 1st Edition

More than 25 years ago, when I was a junior nurse, one of the most useful books I ever bought was a blank notebook in which I wrote notes and procedures on what to do in certain situations. It is not possible to know how to do everything when you are newly qualified, nor is it possible to carry around a complete set of textbooks for quick reference, hence the idea for this book – a pocket-sized handbook containing ideas, principles and guidelines for a number of common and sometimes unexpected situations that you will probably meet in your first year of practice.

I recently had the privilege of working with a group of clinically based practice development nurses, and discussed with them the possibility of writing such a handbook. They were enthusiastic and wanted to take it on as a project. We collected together all the common situations that a newly qualified staff nurse might face, and then volunteered ourselves, or someone else, to write the answers. The result is this guide: more than 70 questions with answers from 14 different specialists. We aimed to produce an answer for each question that could be read in five minutes. This obviously limited the amount of information and rationale that we could include. If you wish to explore any of the subjects in greater depth, you will need to access specialist textbooks. Quay Books is currently producing a complete series of *Fundamental Aspects of Nursing Practice*, which is aimed at senior students and staff nurses.

This book is intended to be a useful handbook for everyday use – do not leave it on your bookshelf in your room. Keep it on the ward, where you can access it easily. At the end of each chapter there is a blank page for you to add useful local information, such as the telephone number of the infection control nurse, or your own notes on a particular procedure. Add notes to this book and make it your own resource. I was asked a question recently by a newly qualified nurse – one that does not appear in this book. It was: 'How can I be a really good nurse?' My answer was simple: 'Find a really good role model and learn from him or her.' I hope you want to be a really good nurse: although it is a difficult job, it is one of the most rewarding careers that anyone can have. Work to the best of your ability, work with enthusiasm, listen to your patients and learn from them. Good luck in your nursing career. I hope you find this handbook useful.

Many thanks to all the contributors for their willingness to share their knowledge and experience in the production of this handbook.

John Fowler
De Montfort University
Leicester 2005

Introduction to the 2nd Edition

I still remember the first few months of my life as a staff nurse, too many years ago to recount! They were one of the most rewarding, yet scary times of my nursing career. Rewarding because all those years of training were now being put into practice. I was given respect, authority, responsibility and, not the least, more pay! And scary for all the same reasons. Looking back I am so grateful to my first ward sister and the other two staff nurses on that ward. I probably did not appreciate at the time how much they supported me, encouraged me and guided me in my early nursing career. Such is the personality of youth, we often to not see and appreciate those around us that are going out of their way to help us. Over the 30 plus years that I have been a nurse I have tried to return some of that support and guidance that was so generously given to me. I hope that this small book is in some way a help to you as you begin your nursing career. Many people have commented how useful they found the first edition and I'm grateful to all the contributors who have yet again given of their time to update and add new sections to this handy little book.

John Fowler
De Montfort University
Leicester 2010

Contributors

Claire Agnew RN(Adult), DipHE Nursing, PGCE, ENB124, ENB 998, Senior Nurse Clinical Practice Development, University of Leicester Hospitals NHS Trust, Leicester

Flo Brett RGN, Previously Clinical Governance Manager, University Hospitals of Leicester NHS Trust, Leicester

Nicola Brooks PG Dip. BSc (Hons), DipHE Nursing, RN, ENB998, ENB931, Senior Lecturer – Adult Nursing, School of Nursing and Midwifery, De Montfort University, Leicester

Deborah Dowsett MA BA(Hons) DPSN RGN, Senior Lecturer - Nursing, School of Nursing and Midwifery, De Montfort University, Leicester

John Fowler PhD MA, BA, DipN, CertED, RGN, RMN, RCNT, RNT, Principal Lecturer - Nursing, School of Nursing and Midwifery, De Montfort University, Leicester

Martyn Geary MA, BA(Hons), RGN, PGCE(FAHE), Senior Lecturer – Palliative Care, School of Nursing and Midwifery, De Montfort University, Leicester

Nigel Goodrich BSc (Hons), DMS, RGN, RMN, Principal Lecturer, School of Nursing and Midwifery, De Montfort University, Leicester

Penny Harrison MA, BSc (Hons), RGN, FETC, CertEd, ENB100, Senior Lecturer – Adult Nursing, School of Nursing and Midwifery, De Montfort University, Leicester

Martin Hopkins MSc BA(Hons) PGCE DipHE RN(Adult), Senior Lecturer, School of Nursing and Midwifery, De Montfort University, Leicester

Karen Jackson BSc (Hons), PG Dip, MMedSci, RGN, RSCN, Senior Lecturer – Children's Nursing, School of Nursing and Midwifery, De Montfort University, Leicester

Tracey Kemmett BSc RGN, Previously Senior Nurse, University Hospitals of Leicester HNS Trust, Leicester

Annie Law MA, PGDAdEd, BA(Hons) DPNS, RGN, RNT, ENB100, N59, ENB931, N14, Practitioner/Lecturer, Directorate of Cancer Services and Clinical Haematology, University Hospitals of Leicester NHS Trust, Leicester

Paul Pleasance EdD, MEd, RGN, ITUCert, PGCE, RNT, ILTM, Head of Quality, Faculty of Health and Life Sciences, De Montfort University, Leicester

Kevin Power MA, BA(Hons), Dip(N), CertEd, RSCN, RGN, Associate Head of School, School of Nursing and Midwifery, De Montfort University, Leicester

Paul Rigby MA, BA(Hons), DipN, DipAdEd, Dip PSI (THORN) RMN, Senior Lecturer – Mental Health, De Montfort University, Leicester

Wendy Taylor BSc (Hons), RGN, In Patient Service Manager – Palliative Care, The Leicestershire and Rutland Hospice, Leicester

Keith Todd RGN, CertEd, ENB199, Senior Lecturer, School of Nursing and Midwifery, De Montfort University, Leicester

Penny Tremayne MSc, PGDE, BSc (Hons), DipN, RGN, Senior Lecturer – Adult Nursing, School of Nursing and Midwifery, De Montfort University, Leicester

Zoe Wilkes MSc BSc (Hons), RGN, RSCN, Assistant Service Manager, Children's Community and Palliative Care Services, Leicester City PCT

CHAPTER 1

Dealing with the unexpected

- How do I deal with difficult questions?
- How do I deal with complaints?
- How do I deal with aggressive patients or relatives?
- What is involved in incident reporting?
- What are my responsibilities in reporting malpractice?
- What can I do about bullying within the organisation?
- What do I do if a patient wants to self-discharge?
- How do I deal with healthcare associated infections?

How do I deal with difficult questions?
Kevin Power

Difficult questions probably fall into two categories: those to which you do not know the answer and those that you are not sure how to answer. The first type is probably relatively easy to deal with. Being honest and telling the questioner that you do not know the answer is the best response. Trying to bluff an answer is fraught with difficulty, as it is always likely that you will be caught out. Many newly qualified staff nurses perceive that other people expect them to 'know everything' because they are qualified, regardless of the length of their experience (Lathlean, 1987; Shand, 1987; Power, 1996; Charnley, 1999; Whitehead 2001). It is also clear that this phenomenon is not restricted to the UK (Cowin and Hengstberger-Sims, 2006). However, it is unreasonable to expect anyone to know the answer to all the questions that may be asked. There should be no shame in admitting that you are temporarily at a loss for an answer. Obviously you will promise to find out the answer or find someone who can give that answer, and it is important to keep that promise.

The second type of difficult question is altogether more challenging. This type of question may fall into one of two categories. The answer may be rather complex and the difficulty here is making sure that your explanation is easily understood by the questioner. The best way to approach such situations is to build up a personal 'thesaurus' of everyday words that mean the same as or explain technical jargon. For example, a patient may ask what a lesion is, as the doctor mentioned this to them. This word can have a variety of meanings, ranging from an innocent wart to a potentially devastating cancer.

Case study 1

Amit Shah had recently been diagnosed as having leukaemia. He said to the nurse caring for him that the doctor had explained the disease to him but he did not really understand what the doctor was saying as he had used some long unintelligible words. The nurse asked some basic questions of Amit in order to establish how much he did know. She then gathered pens and paper and drew a picture using an analogy of opposing armies fighting a battle to explain how the disease happened and progressed. The combination of the use of lay language and pictures enabled Amit to understand much more clearly what was going on in his body.

Having a ready response that can explain such words in lay terms will enable you to ensure that patients or relatives understand their care and treatment (see Case Study 1).

The second category of question that you may not be sure how to answer is probably a question that has an ethical component. An example of this would be when a patient asks what is wrong with him or her, when you know a decision has been made by the multidisciplinary team not to reveal the true diagnosis at this point in the patient's care. The Code (Nursing and Midwifery Council (NMC), 2008a: 2) states:

You must share with people, in a way they can understand, the information they want or need to know about their health.

You must uphold people's rights to be fully involved in decisions about their care.

Some have argued that physicians (and by extension any health professional) should '...cultivate lying as a fine art' (Collins, 1988) in order to bolster the hopes of patients, who may be seriously ill, and prevent them from losing the will to live. Whether everyone could learn to lie effectively and control their facial expression is a moot point. Jackson (2001) is unequivocal in her condemnation of all lies, whether trivial or serious. I always advise my students to avoid all lies in their practice. Anything that has the potential to reduce a patient's or relative's trust in nurses should probably be avoided; lying is fairly certain to reduce that trust and all lies have the potential to be discovered (see Case Study 2).

Generally, if a person asks a question it is because he or she wants to hear the answer. When a patient has a serious condition with a poor prognosis,

---

Case study 2

Sally Dent, the mother of 5-year-old Ben, insisted that nurses did not tell her son that he would have any pain following some relatively minor surgery. No amount of persuasion would shift Sally's view and she remained insistent. The nurses decided that they would accede to Sally's wish as they reasoned she knew her son best. Ben did ask, 'Will it hurt?', and the nurse kept silent when his mum assured him that it would not. After returning from theatre, Ben, despite having received analgesia as part of the anaesthetic, was in some discomfort although not significant pain. He became very distressed, shouting at the nurses that they had lied to him as it did hurt. The rest of his short stay in hospital was difficult as he was unwilling for the nurses to do much for him.

---

many staff nurses tell me that they have the feeling the patient already knows and is merely seeking confirmation. Thus the honest and truthful answer may not be a shock to the patient. That does not mean that the patient will not become upset, and you must prepare yourself to provide appropriate comfort in such situations. There is, of course, a potential risk of upsetting other members of the team by revealing the truth after a decision has been made to withhold a diagnosis. A professional judgement has to be made whether or not to reveal the truth.

There are also ways of addressing such questions without the need to resort to lying. One could truthfully answer: 'I am afraid I cannot answer that question at the moment.' This does run the risk of patients then saying: 'Why, because you don't know or because you don't want to tell me?' A reasonable response could then be that you are not the best person to ask and that you will arrange for them to speak to someone who can answer their questions effectively.

How do I deal with complaints?
Kevin Power

In the report for 2007–2008, the Parliamentary and Health Service Ombudsman stated that complaints about care are often aggravated by the way in which complaints were dealt with. 'Poor complaint handling by NHS bodies and individuals was a recurrent theme across our health investigations in 2007–08' (Parliamentary and Health Service Ombudsman, 2009: 36). The problem with some complaints is that they may begin as minor issues, but, if not dealt with properly, can become a major confrontation. The way a nurse deals with a complaint at the very beginning of the process can thus have an effect on the whole course of that complaint.

The simplest way to deal with complaints is to prevent them occurring in the first place. Be on the lookout for signs that a patient or relative is getting irritated; do not wait for the complaint – ask whether there is a problem. I remember sitting completing a duty rota and overhearing a father sounding cross on the telephone outside the ward office. It was clear that something was wrong. When I went to investigate, it seemed that no-one had told him what was going on with his young daughter, who had been admitted as an emergency, and he had an important business meeting to attend. When I asked the staff caring for the child to explain what the delay was and the likely timeframe for her admission, he was able to make some arrangements with his work and became much calmer.

If this situation had been ignored it is highly likely that a formal complaint would have been lodged. However, it is unlikely that the health service is going to please all of the people all of the time, no matter how high your personal standards of care or how good your communication skills. Patients and relatives may be in pain or anxious and certainly in a strange environment. Additionally, as staff are under pressure because of high workloads and staff shortages, there are always likely to be complaints of some kind or another.

Most NHS trusts actively seek feedback from patients and service users as part of clinical governance (Robotham, 2001). This may enable trusts to forestall complaints through improvements to the service. It may also encourage more people to complain. Each trust will have protocols and policies in place for dealing with formal complaints and you should be familiar with these. Let us focus for the purposes of this section on those situations where a relative or patient makes a verbal complaint to you. Think of a time when you have complained about something:

- What was the cause of the complaint?
- Who did you complain to?

- How was the complaint dealt with?
- How did this make you feel?

Most complaints are fairly mundane, but no matter how trivial to the member of staff, all are important to the complainant. When thinking about times when I have complained, the response of the person I have complained to has had a great impact on how far I wanted to take the complaint and the level of redress I expected. So how do you, as the nurse receiving a verbal complaint, respond? The Wilson Report (Department of Health, 1994) identified several lessons from the private sector.

- Complainants want an apology, even if the organisation was not at fault: This does not mean accepting responsibility for the problem. Just saying sorry that the person feels there is a problem may at least show that you are acknowledging their concerns.
- Complainants want a speedy response: Show that you are willing to take action immediately, even if it is just to make the time to listen to the complaint. This is difficult when you are busy, but making the complainant wait or passing them on to a more senior member of staff can escalate the situation (see also Robotham, 2001; Parliamentary and Health Service Ombudsman, 2009).
- Complainants want a reassurance that the organisation is taking the matter seriously and will try to prevent a recurrence: Do inform complainants what you intend to do about their complaint and how the trust will respond.
- Complainants do not want to be told:
  - that rules were being followed, so the organisation was right all along,
  - that they made a mistake, so it is their own fault,
  - detailed explanations of why a problem arose, which come across as an excuse for poor services.
- It should be an objective to resolve as many complaints as possible at the first point of contact: It is important that when a person complains, you try to handle it yourself in the first instance. Find out whether your employer provides training on complaints handling and ask to be sent for some. This can mean that you are better prepared to deal with complaints as they arise. However, if, after listening carefully, it becomes clear that you cannot resolve the issue or that it is a serious matter, you should inform the complainant about how to take the matter further.

If this is the first time you have had to deal with a complaint, make sure you seek support from your senior nurse or duty manager. You will not be expected to deal with a complaint by yourself, and more senior staff will expect to be involved. Also, no matter how competently you deal with a complaint, some people will not be satisfied until they have spoken to someone 'in authority'. If your situation seems to be heading this way, do not see it as a failure – swallow your pride and call in a suitable member of staff.

Finally, do not forget to record the complaint and the action you took. Even if you feel that the complaint was dealt with immediately, the complainant may want to take things further at a later date. Clear records of the complaint, times and dates and the outcome will be vital if a formal investigation takes place.

How do I deal with aggressive patients or relatives?
Kevin Power

There are occasions when a person will not complain in a reasonable manner but becomes verbally or physically aggressive. People may kick, punch, slap or bite, they may make verbal insults or threats or make threatening gestures. All of these are considered to come under the broad heading of aggression (Garnham, 2001). As with many things, prevention is better than cure. It is important to be aware of the factors that may lead to aggression and act to reduce them. Keeping people informed is particularly important as frustration can arise from anxiety and fear of the unknown, especially in strange environments such as hospitals. This may be made worse by the illness itself and the feelings of lack of control that patients or relatives may feel. For example, if there is time to be spent waiting to be seen by a member of staff it is important to keep going back every so often to apologise for the delay and explain why they may need to wait. In this situation, always be honest about the delay and do not try to invent an excuse, as this, if discovered, will only make the situation worse.

Spotting aggression before it happens and doing something to prevent it occurring is the ideal situation. However, this is not always possible, especially if the aggression is a result of alcohol, drugs or some altered state of consciousness and/or perception.

How should I deal with aggression when it happens?

Garnham (2001) recommends the use of the firefighting model to deal with aggression. Basically this means identifying the elements that need to be present for a violent incident to occur and removing one of those elements. The four elements are:

- A target.
- A weapon.
- A trigger.
- A state of arousal.

Removing the target will usually mean that someone needs to leave the area. If it is another patient or relative you must gently persuade them that it is best to move away from the situation. Care needs to be taken here to ensure that you do not make yourself into the target. If you are the target for the aggression, withdrawing from the situation is likely to resolve the immediate problem, but may just mean that someone else becomes the target.

Removing a weapon that is being used can be impossible if it is a fist or a foot, and inadvisable if a knife or heavy object. You should on no account attempt to restrain or disarm someone unless you have received specific training to do this. You might ask the person to put the weapon down.

The trigger for the aggression may be easily removed if it is the behaviour of another person. But if the trigger is frustration over waiting times or the way that someone has just spoken to the aggressor, this cannot be removed once it has caused the aggression. Sometimes the trigger will seem to be trivial, but you need to remember that patients and relatives might already be in a heightened state of arousal as a result of the admission.

You may be able to reduce the state of arousal of the aggressive person. It is important to maintain eye contact (Garnham, 2001), but not to appear threatening by trying to stare the aggressor down. Speak calmly and be aware of body posture. You need to be assertive without being aggressive yourself.

Without being patronising, do acknowledge the source of the frustration and anger. This can be done by simply saying something like, 'I accept that this situation is frustrating for you but...'. Let the aggressor know that their behaviour is making you uncomfortable or frightened (Garnham, 2001). You might try to appease the person by suggesting that you may be able to do something to resolve the situation. However, do not promise anything that cannot be delivered. For example, do not promise that you will get someone more senior to address the problem unless you can be fairly sure that the senior person will take some action.

You may not be able to do anything about the state of arousal of the aggressive person if he or she is under the influence of alcohol or drugs or in a confused state. If all else fails or you feel that you cannot personally deal with the situation, you should call for assistance. If you work in the community and are in a patient's house, you should leave the moment you feel in danger. If there are other people in the house who you feel might be attacked by the aggressive person, you should call the police.

Whatever the outcome of the situation, you should of course make clear and accurate records of what transpired, the action you took and the outcome of the incident (see below for incident reporting). Ferns and Chojnacka (2005) identified a number of potential barriers to effective reporting of aggression towards staff in the NHS and it is important to be aware of these and seek help in overcoming them to ensure effective reporting of incidents.

What is involved in incident reporting?

Kevin Power

According to the Government's Chief Medical Officer, one in 10 hospital patients suffers some accidental harm (*British Journal of Nursing*, 2002). Your immediate response to the incident is important. Clearly the priority is to ensure that anyone who is actually hurt receives prompt attention for their injuries. Green (2001) notes some confusion regarding how to respond when an incident occurs. Where an incident occurs that may lead to a claim against a nurse, the Royal College of Nursing (RCN) (2009) advises:

> *Remember that you should never admit liability for an incident or submit any written statement about it until you have taken advice from the RCN.*

It is likely that other professional indemnity schemes will contain similar advice. This advice is contrary to the stated aims for the management of clinical risk in the NHS (Green, 2001). One of these aims is for staff to be able to listen, apologise and learn from their mistakes.

So what do you do when faced with an incident? Do you apologise or seek union advice? Green (2001) advises that a nurse should not rush to apologise for an incident, but should record the facts, ensure that the line manager is made aware of the incident promptly, and cooperate with the complaints procedure. Green (2001) suggests that completion of the investigation may be an appropriate point at which to apologise without compromising any indemnity insurance you may have.

It is clear that all incidents leading to harm, whether minor or major, must be reported (Department of Health, 2001). Any incidents that nearly led to harm (near misses) must also be reported. Each employer will have local systems for reporting incidents and near misses, and you should be familiar with the system in operation in your own area.

There are minimum requirements for the recording of incidents. These are listed in the box below.

Essential details to record in an incident report

- The fact that the examination was carried out
- Whether any injury was apparent
- Any advice given to the injured person

What do I write?

When writing the record it is important to note clear and unambiguous facts.

- What you saw or what others say they saw, not what you or they think happened.

For example, if a patient falls, do not write: 'Mrs Smith seemed to have fallen out of bed.' Instead, write: 'Mrs Smith was found lying on the floor next to her bed'. You can record what someone says, for example: 'Mrs Smith stated that she fell out of bed.'

Where you do record what someone says, it important to make it clear that it is someone else's words by enclosing the statement in quotation marks. You should also write down the events in chronological order as this can help to clarify precisely what happened. Any witnesses to the event should make a statement, and if the witness is another patient, a relative or a junior member of staff, they may need advice on how to write what happened to ensure that they also report facts rather than what they think happened.

If any person was injured or there is a suspicion of injury as a result of the incident, a doctor should examine that person. You should ensure that the doctor carrying out such an examination records:

- What happened (event or near miss description, severity of actual or potential harm, people and equipment involved)?
- Where did it happen (location/specialty)?
- When did it happen (date and time)?
- How did it happen (immediate or proximate cause(s))?
- Why did it happen (underlying or root cause(s))?
- What action was taken or proposed (immediate and longer term)?
- What impact did the event have (harm to the organisation, the patient, others)?
- What factors did, or could have, minimised the impact of the event?

(Department of Health, 2001)

What are my responsibilities in reporting malpractice?
Kevin Power

There are two types of situation that may lead you to report malpractice. The first relates specifically to those whose names appear on a professional register, such as nurses and doctors, and is usually termed professional misconduct. The second is malpractice by anyone within the care area or concerns about poor standards.

Professional misconduct

Nurses are advised to discuss any concerns they have about a registered colleague with their employer in the first instance (NMC, 2008b). *Table 1.1* lists the most common types of professional misconduct reported to the NMC.

Therefore, you need to be sure of your facts and give a clear factual account of your concerns, that means stating what has actually occurred rather than what you suspect may have occurred. If you can get other witnesses to support your concerns, all the better. If there are no other witnesses, record all the facts including date and time and precisely what you observed. Remember to write down what you saw, not what you think happened.

Table 1.1. The most common types of professional misconduct allegations reported to the NMC		
	2006–2007	2007–2008
Dishonesty*	19.23%	17.32%
Patient abuse (physical, sexual, verbal, inappropriate relationship)	17.09%	14.30%
Failure to maintain adequate records	7.48%	10.37%
Maladministration of drugs	10.47%	9.87%
Neglect of basic care	10.04%	9.16%
Unsafe clinical practice	7.48%	7.75%
Failure to collaborate with colleagues	4.06%	6.95%
Colleague abuse (physical, sexual, verbal, inappropriate relationship)	4.27%	2.72%
Failure to report incidents	3.42%	2.62%
Failure to act in an emergency	3.21%	1.91%
Pornography - adult	2.35%	1.01%
*Dishonesty includes theft, fraud, and false claim to registration, claiming sick pay fraudulently, falsification of records and dishonesty about previous employment and misappropriation of drugs.** NMC, 2008c		

Many nurses are afraid to report poor standards and malpractice because of the potential for recriminations and possibly even loss of their job (O'Dowd, 2002). Certainly, students that I teach often say they would be unlikely to complain about poor standards of care that they witness, out of fear of being failed by their assessor as a reprisal. This culture of fear of reprisals seems to persist for qualified nurses (Nazarko, 1998; Health Which, 1999; Wallis, 2001; Ferns and Chojnacka, 2005). This appears to remain the case despite the enactment of the Public Interest Disclosure Act 1998, which protects the whistleblower if victimised or dismissed as a result of disclosing malpractice.

To whom should I report malpractice?

Under the Public Interest Disclosure Act 1998, protection from victimisation and dismissal by an employer is given to those who speak out against any malpractice. Areas covered by the Public Interest Disclosure Act 1998 are listed in the box below. However, this does not give carte blanche for anyone to go directly to the press with a complaint. All other reasonable attempts should be made to rectify a situation before going to the media. You should first raise any concerns internally with your employer, and if no progress is made you may take those concerns to a prescribed regulator; only then, if no progress is made, should concerns be raised externally to your employer. You are, however, allowed to seek legal advice and still be protected by the Act. If you decide to go to the media in the first instance, there is likely to be less protection from some sanctions, such as dismissal by your employer (RCN, 2004).

Areas covered by the Public Interest Disclosure Act

- A criminal act
- A failure to comply with legal obligation (including negligence, breach of contract, including contract of employment, and breach of administrative law)
- A miscarriage of justice
- Danger to health and safety
- Damage to the environment
- An attempt to cover up any of these

Malpractice covered by the Public Interest Disclosure Act 1998

Concerns should first be raised with your employer, such as your line manager, senior colleague or supervisor. For example, if you are a staff nurse then you should raise the issue with the charge nurse or more senior nurse. If the person you have concerns about is your manager and you work in the NHS, you have the right to raise concerns with the trust board, the health authority or even a health minister (RCN, 2004).

Prescribed regulator

If you work in the independent sector, such as a nursing home or private hospital, concerns can be raised with a prescribed regulator. Regulators include the Health and Safety Executive, the Inland Revenue, the Audit Commission and the local authority. You may also report concerns to a prescribed regulator if you feel that those concerns have not been acted upon by an NHS employer.

Legal adviser

Should you need independent and confidential advice about a concern of malpractice, disclosures to a legal adviser are protected under the Act. This means that you can seek a legal opinion without being accused of breaching confidentiality.

Reporting malpractice externally

The Act does allow for reporting of malpractice to the police, media, MPs etc. under exceptional circumstances, i.e. where one of the following conditions is satisfied:

- Reasonable belief that the person reporting malpractice would be victimised if he or she raised the matter internally or with a prescribed person.
- There is no prescribed person, and reasonable belief that the evidence would be concealed or destroyed.
- The concern had already been raised with the employer or prescribed person. (RCN, 2004)

It may also be advisable to seek advice from a representative of your union. However, the law does give the greatest protection for internal disclosure, which includes reports made to Government ministers. If you decided to take your concerns to the media before raising them with your employer, the Act would provide less protection from dismissal than if you had used the institution's grievance procedures. There is a good deal of useful advice on reporting malpractice on the Public Concern at Work website (http://www.pcaw.co.uk). The box below lists some useful tips suggested on this website.

Whistle-blowing advice

- Stay calm
- Remember that you are a witness, and not a complainant
- Think about the risks and outcomes before you act
- Let the facts speak for themselves - don't make ill-considered allegations
- Remember that you may be mistaken or that there may be an innocent or good explanation
- Do not become a private detective
- Recognise that you may not be thanked

(Public Concern at Work, 2009)

What can I do about bullying within the organisation?
Kevin Power

Bullying is increasingly being recognised as a problem. Indeed, an RCN survey revealed that up to one in six nurses is subject to bullying at work (Pearce, 2001). If you are being bullied, you will generally want it to stop. However, as a nurse you probably also have a professional duty to take action if you are aware that someone else is being bullied. Although the NMC Code of Professional Conduct (NMC, 2008a) does not make explicit mention of bullying, it does state that there is a duty to report circumstances in the care environment that could jeopardise standards of practice. It would be hard to imagine anyone delivering a high standard of care if they were subject to bullying. There is probably also a duty placed on you by your employer through local policies which outline action that should be taken if you are aware of bullying. How do you recognise when you or another member of staff is being bullied? It is not always obvious when you are being bullied. Howells-Johnson (2000) defines bullying as persistent unwelcome behaviour, such as:

- Unwarranted or invalid criticism.
- Nit-picking.
- Fault finding.
- Exclusion.
- Isolation of another.
- Singling someone out.
- Treating someone differently.
- Shouting at someone.
- Humiliating someone.
- Excessive monitoring of someone's work performance.

Other examples might include making unreasonable work demands on a person and inciting others to hold a negative opinion of someone.

What should you do?

The first thing to do is to recognise bullying behaviour for what it is. There can be no excuse for it, especially in the workplace. Any criticism of your or anyone else's performance should be constructive and based on facts, not destructive and based on conjecture or mere opinion. As with much of what is discussed in this chapter, record what is happening. According to Grove (2000) it is not the incident itself that necessarily counts, but the frequency and the regularity with which it happens. White (2002a) also suggests talking to colleagues about the bullying, as you might not be the only one. Alternatively, if it is not you that is being bullied, but a colleague, talking to others may reveal several team members who do not like the situation and are prepared to support you in taking action against the bully.

Your trust or employer should have anti-bullying policies in place. Find out what they are and use them to take action. Dimond (2002) points out that your employer has a legal duty under health and safety law to protect employees from bullying. Additionally, under Article 3 of the Human Rights Act 1998, you have the right to freedom from inhuman and degrading treatment. It is inhuman and degrading to bully someone and the employer has a clear duty to prevent this abuse of human rights. You also have legal protection under the Public Interest Disclosure Act 1998 if you blow the whistle and report an employer for bullying (see section on reporting malpractice on page 11).

You should be aware of the potentially detrimental effects that bullying can have on your health and should seek medical advice if you feel that your health is affected. If you are off sick as a result of bullying, record it in the accident book at work. If necessary, you can take out a grievance against the bully through your employer's grievance procedures. Human resources or personnel departments should be able to give advice and support in this.

Your union representative should also be able to offer advice and guidance on handling the situation. Several case studies of bullying reported in the press indicate that the victims felt embarrassed about being a victim and suffered in silence until they were driven out of their job. The key is not to suffer alone but to share your feelings with others and report bullying behaviour. Grove (2000) goes as far as suggesting that if the bully is aggressive in public, you should get a solicitor's letter sent to the bully with regard to the slander or defamation of character. The most important thing is not to allow the bully to win by forcing a change in your behaviour or moving jobs. Not only will your self-esteem take a serious blow, but the bully is likely to move on to another target. You should not have to pay the price for someone else's unacceptable behaviour.

What do I do if a patient wants to self-discharge?
Kevin Power

All patients, unless detained under the Mental Health Act 1983, are voluntary and cannot be kept in hospital or a nursing/residential home against their will. You have a professional duty to ensure the safety and wellbeing of people who lack the capacity to make decisions for themselves. Thus, if a person lacks that capacity and is intending to self-discharge, it may be necessary to consider seeking a psychiatric referral.

If, on the other hand, there is no evidence of any lack of capacity, any person over the age of 18 years has the right to decide for themselves whether to accept or reject medical advice, including whether to remain in hospital. Merely wanting to discharge oneself against medical advice is not evidence of lack of capacity to make a rational decision.

It is preferable that persons wishing to discharge themselves sign a written declaration that they are taking self-discharge against medical advice. Your employer should have forms for this specific purpose. However, there is no legal requirement that the patient actually signs the form. So what can you do if a patient decides to self-discharge and refuses to sign the declaration/form? Recording the event is imperative. Some indication of the patient's reasons for self-discharge might be helpful. However, the essential facts that must be recorded are the time and date the patient left. It is also important to record any advice that was given to the patient by yourself or anyone else.

What advice should you give?

If the patient is willing to listen, you should consider informing them:

- Why it is best to remain in hospital.
- The potential health consequences of taking self-discharge at that point in their care.
- That they should inform their own GP.
- That the consultant will probably inform their GP.
- How to continue their care at home.
- When to seek help from a medical practitioner.
- The telephone number of NHS Direct.
- The hospital/ward contact number.

It might also be useful to consider producing a leaflet outlining general advice regarding self-discharge if your institution does not already have one. You should, of course, ensure that, if the medical staff do not already know, they are informed immediately of the situation.

How do I deal with healthcare associated infections?
Kevin Power

Antibiotic-resistant bacteria are a constant worry in the health service. The media regularly report outbreaks of 'superbugs'. So how should you tackle this problem? Methicillin-resistant Staphylococcus aureus (MRSA) and Clostridium difficile (C. diff) are the two causative agents that are of most concern but this should not obscure the fact that there are many potential sources of infection in healthcare institutions and the home. There is helpful specific advice on the Department of Health website which deals specifically with both MRSA and C.diff.

MRSA

The following is taken from the Department of Health's (2007a) advice sheet and more detailed information is held on its website.

- To reduce the likelihood of spreading infection, you should always wash your hands or use an antibacterial hand rub after you have had any physical contact with a patient – whether or not the patient has a wound. Remember that healthcare workers can be carriers of the bacteria even if they are not infected themselves.
- You should also encourage patients to wash their hands after using the toilet and before and after eating.
- If you suspect infection, there is a simple test which involves taking a swab or other sample from the suspected site of infection and sending it for laboratory analysis. Also check patients' antibiotics to make sure their treatment is appropriate for MRSA.
- If patients are infected, always use gloves when treating them and consider moving them away from other patients to help prevent the bacteria spreading.
- In high-risk situations (e.g. patients admitted for major surgery, such as a hip replacement or heart surgery) if pre-screening shows MRSA carriage, decontamination with skin and nose treatment is recommended before patients are operated on.

Clostridium difficile

The following advice is taken from the Department of Health's (2009) website:

- All staff should apply the following mnemonic protocol (SIGHT) when managing suspected potentially infectious diarrhoea:

S: Suspect that a case may be infective where there is no clear alternative cause for diarrhoea.

I: Isolate the patient and consult with the infection control team (ICT) while determining the cause of the diarrhoea.

G: Gloves and aprons must be used for all contacts with the patient and his or her environment.

H: Hand washing with soap and water should be carried out before and after each contact with the patient and the patient's environment.

T: Test the stool for toxin, by sending a specimen immediately.

Further guidance is offered by the Department of Health's (2007b) publication

- Always wash your hands after you have had any physical contact with a patient. Do not rely solely on alcohol gel as this does not kill C. difficile spores.
- To keep cases of C. difficile down, healthcare workers should look to avoid prescribing broad spectrum antibiotics, as far as possible, so that patients' natural protection is not weakened
- If you suspect infection, there is a simple diagnostic test that can be done on a sample of diarrhoeal faeces to see if C. difficile toxins are present. It gives a result within a few hours. In outbreaks, or for surveillance of the different strains circulating in the population, C. difficile can be cultured from faeces and the isolates sent to the Anaerobe Reference Laboratory (National Public Health Service, Wales; Microbiology, Cardiff) or HPA Regional Laboratories for typing and testing for susceptibility to antibiotics.
- Infected patients should be isolated and healthcare workers dealing with them should wear gloves and aprons, especially when dealing with bedpans, etc.
- Environments should be kept clean at all times. Where there are cases of C. difficile infection, a disinfectant containing chlorine or other sporicidal agent should be used to reduce environmental contamination with the spores.

The Department of Health (2006) provides specific guidance for nursing and residential homes in dealing with healthcare associated infections.

Final points

Remember that if a patient cannot mobilise and is confined to a side room with a label of 'infectious', he or she is probably going to feel isolated and possibly stigmatised. You can help the patient by encouraging visitors to stagger the times of their visits. Make sure that the patient understands his or her condition and is not isolated unless absolutely essential. All trusts will have an infection control nurse or team, which will be an invaluable source of information and support to the ward staff and the patient.

References

British Journal of Nursing (2002) One in 10 hospital patients suffer some form of harm. *British Journal of Nursing* **11**(12): 796

Charnley E (1999) Occupational stress in the newly qualified staff nurse. *Nursing Standard* **13**(29): 33–36

Collins J (1988) Should doctors tell the truth? In: Callaghan J (Ed) *Ethical Issues in Modern Medicine*. Oxford University Press, Oxford

Cowin L, Hengstberger-Sims C (2006) New graduate nurse self-concept and retention: A longitudinal study. *International Journal of Nursing Studies* **43**(1): 59–70

Department of Health (1994) *Being Heard: The report of a review committee on NHS complaints procedures* (Wilson Report). HMSO, London

Department of Health (2001) *Building a Safer NHS for Patients: Implementing an organisation with a memory*. Department of Health, London

Department of Health (2006) *Essential steps to safe, clean care: Reducing healthcare-associated infections*. From: http://www.dh.gov.uk/en/ Publicationsandstatistics/Publications/PublicationsPolicyAndGuidance/ DH_4136212

Department of Health (2007a) *A simple guide to MRSA*. DH London

Department of Health (2007b) *A simple guide to C. Difficile*. DH. London

Department of Health (2009) *Clostridium difficile infection: How to deal with the problem*. DH. London

Dimond B (2002) Workplace stress and bullying: Liabilities of the employer. *British Journal of Nursing* **11**(10) 699–701

Ferns T, Chojnacka I (2005) Reporting incidents of violence and aggression towards NHS staff. *Nursing Standard* **19**(38): 51–6

Garnham P (2001) Understanding and dealing with anger, aggression and violence. *Nursing Standard* **16**(6): 37–42

Green C (2001) Benefiting from the end of blame culture. *Professional Nurse* **16**(7 Suppl): S3–S4

Grove J (2000) Survival and resistance. *Nursing Times* **96**(18): 26–8

Health Which? (1999) Blowing the whistle. *Health Which?* April: 16–17

Howells-Johnson J (2000) Verbal abuse. *British Journal of Perioperative Nursing* **10**(10): 508–11

Jackson J (2001) *Truth, Trust and Medicine*. Routledge, London

Lathlean J (1987) Are you prepared to be a staff nurse? *Nursing Times* **83**(36): 25–7

Lomas C (2009) Nurses must receive sufficient continence education and training. *Nursing Times* **105**(21): 32–3

Madeo M, Roodhouse AJ (2009) Reducing the risks associated with urinary catheters. *Nursing Standard* **23**(29): 47–55

McBride J, Knight D, Piper J, Smith G (2005) Long-term effect of introducing an early warning score on respiratory rate charting on general wards.

Resuscitation **65**: 41–4

Nazarko L (1998) Breaking the silence. *Elder Care* **10**(3): 44

Nursing and Midwifery Council (2008a) *The Code: Standards of Conduct, Performance and Ethics for Nurses and Midwives*. Nursing and Midwifery Council, London

Nursing and Midwifery Council (2008b) *Environment of care advice sheet*. Nursing and Midwifery Council London. Online at http://www.Nursing and Midwifery Council-uk. org/aDisplayDocument.aspx?documentID=3987

Nursing and Midwifery Council (2008c) *Fitness to Practise Annual Report 1 April 2007 to 31 March 2008*. Nursing and Midwifery Council, London

O'Dowd A (2002) Is legislation protecting nurses who blow the whistle? *Nursing Times* **98**(46): 10–11

Parliamentary and Health Service Ombudsman (2009) *Annual Report 2007–08*. The Stationary Office, London

Pearce L (2001) Bully at work. *Nursing Standard* **15**(27): 14–15

Power K (1996) First time practice as a children's nurse: A phenomenological inquiry. Unpublished dissertation. De Montfort University, Leicester

Public concern at work (2009) *How do I blow the whistle?* Online at http://www.pcaw.co.uk/FAQ_individuals.htm

Robotham M (2001) How to handle complaints. *Nursing Times* **97**(30): 25–8

Royal College of Nursing (2004) *Blowing the Whistle*. RCN, London

Royal College of Nursing (2009) Legal help. http://www.rcn.org.uk/support/legal [accessed 09.06.2009]

Shand M (1987) Unreasonable expectations? *Nursing Times* **83**(36): 28–30

Wallis L (2001) Protecting the whistleblower. *Nursing Standard* **13**(47): 16–17

White C (2002) The enemy within. *Nursing Times* **98**(44): 12–13

Whitehead J (2001) Newly qualified staff nurses' perceptions of the role transition. *British Journal of Nursing* **10**(5): 330–9

Notes

CHAPTER 2

Clinical nursing skills

- How can I recognise an acutely ill patient?
- What do I need to know about cardiorespiratory arrest?
- How do I carry out basic life support?
- What are the principles of preparing patients for tests and investigations?
- What is a syringe driver?
- How do I monitor central venous pressure?
- What do I need to know about different wound dressings?
- What does an aseptic technique involve?
- What is involved in catheterisation and catheter care?
- How can I promote continence?
- What do I need to know about pressure areas?
- How do I help my patients meet their nutritional needs?
- What are the principles of caring for patients with wound drains?
- How do I look after a nasogastric or gastric tube?
- What is the nursing management of intravenous therapy?

How can I recognise an acutely ill patient?
Martin Hopkins

Patients are admitted to hospital for a multitude of reasons and due to complex factors such as co-morbidity, age and underlying diagnosis are at a high risk of becoming acutely ill (Armitage et al, 2007). It is the responsibility of the registered nurse not only to recognise an acutely ill patient, but also to intervene and provide appropriate emergency care.

Acute deterioration of a patient's condition is usually preceded by a decline in physiological parameters (Subbe et al, 2001). It is therefore essential that all registered nurses can recognise deterioration in patients' observations as well as the physical appearance of the patient.

As a nurse you need to use all observations available to you, including visual observation of the patient. It is a good idea to remember that if your patient *looks* unwell, he or she probably *is* unwell. All patients should have a full set of observations completed upon arrival to hospital including respiration rate, pulse, temperature, blood pressure, level of consciousness and oxygen saturations (National Institute of Health and Clinical Excellence,

2007). This will give you a baseline to work from, with any fluctuation in these highlighting potential changes in your patient's condition.

Patient deterioration

Patients can deteriorate over different time periods dependant upon the underlying cause for the deterioration. The documentation of regular observations can identify the early deterioration of your patient, but these are not recorded as often as would be liked (Resuscitation Council (UK), 2005c). Once you have identified a change in your patient's condition, it can be difficult to know what to do next. Any change should be documented and reported to a senior nursing or medical colleague immediately. Many clinical areas now use a physiological track and trigger system as recommended by National Institute of Health and Clinical Excellence (NICE) (2007) to identify the early deterioration of patients' conditions. These systems are commonly known as Early Warning Scores (EWS) or Modified Early Warning Scores (MEWS). The MEWS system allocates points to the physical observation depending on how deranged from the normal parameters they are (Resuscitation Council (UK), 2005). The overall score informs the nurse of the risk status of the patient, either actual or potential, and informs them of a plan of care. The MEWS systems not only alert the nursing staff to changes in the patient's physical parameters but also inform the nurse of the necessary actions to take. This ensures the patient receives appropriate early intervention to prevent further deterioration or death.

The use of the MEWS systems improves patient monitoring and the documentation of observations (McBride et al, 2005), but has also been proven to identify patients who are at high risk of deterioration and allow for early intervention by medical staff (Goldhill and McNarry, 2004).

The level of observation patients require depends on their underlying diagnosis, initial observations, clinical area of care and their MEWS. However, it is important to realise that the physical observations required to calculate a patient's MEWS depends on the clinical area the patient is in, e.g. medical ward, surgical ward, etc.

It is important to note that the patient may look unwell but have normal observations. This may be due to their compensatory mechanism and therefore if you have any concerns for the wellbeing of your patient, always report to a senior colleague. Never rely on one system alone, this would be like relying only on a patient's pulse to monitor his or her condition and not recognising the patient has stopped breathing. It may be that you have recognised your patient's deteriorating condition utilising your observations and MEWS, but your patient may deteriorate rapidly and suffer cardiac arrest.

What do I need to know about cardiorespiratory arrest?

Martin Hopkins and Keith Todd

Cardiorespiratory arrest may be a result of a primary airway, breathing or cardiovascular problem (Resuscitation Council (UK), 2002) but resuscitation should be attempted if the patient is 'unconscious or unresponsive and not breathing normally' (Resuscitation Council (UK), 2005a). The cardiovascular and respiratory systems function together to achieve perfusion and oxygenation of body cells, and in this sense are interdependent. Indeed, both systems need to receive a constant supply of oxygenated blood. This interaction and interdependence can have consequences for both systems if either is compromised. For example:

- Hypoxaemia may cause myocardial ischaemia which may lead to myocardial infarction and cardiac arrest.
- Serious illness, e.g. sepsis, may cause increased oxygen consumption and increased respiratory workload.
- Heart failure may be a consequence of respiratory failure and vice versa (Resuscitation Council (UK), 2002).

Whenever we talk of a cardiac arrest or a respiratory arrest, we are referring to a physiological system failure that potentially will affect both systems and cause cardiorespiratory arrest.

Causes of cardiorespiratory arrest

Jevon (2002) and the Resuscitation Council (UK) (2002) state that cardiac arrest can be caused by a primary airway, respiratory or cardiac problem, or may occur secondary to any life-threatening illness that compromises the airway, breathing or circulation. Both Jevon and the Resuscitation Council categorise the causes of cardiorespiratory arrest under three principal headings:

Airway obstruction
Airway obstruction may be partial or complete and be caused by:

- Vomit.
- Blood.
- Foreign body, e.g. food, teeth or dentures.
- Direct trauma to the face or throat causing oedema to mouth or pharynx and occlusion from teeth, blood, etc.

- Burns causing laryngeal oedema.
- Unconsciousness and central nervous system depression, e.g. following head injury, metabolic disorder such as diabetic ketoacidosis or hypoglycaemia, alcohol ingestion, opioid analgesics and general anaesthetics.
- Epiglottitis.
- Pharyngeal swelling, e.g. caused by infection or oedema.
- Laryngospasm caused by inflammation or anaphylaxis.
- Bronchospasm or bronchial secretions.
- Pulmonary oedema.

Complete airway obstruction rapidly leads to cardiac arrest. Partial obstruction often precedes complete obstruction and if not resolved within a few minutes may result in cerebral and other vital organ injury leading to cardiac arrest (Nolan et al, 2005).

Respiratory or breathing problems

Respiratory or breathing problems leading to respiratory/cardiopulmonary arrest include:

- Pulmonary disorders, such as:
  - Asthma
  - Pulmonary oedema
  - Pulmonary embolus (PE)
  - Infection
  - Aspiration of gastric contents or blood from trauma
  - Exacerbation of chronic obstructive pulmonary disease (COPD)
  - Acute respiratory distress syndrome
  - Haemothorax
  - Pneumothorax or tension pneumothorax (spontaneous or as a result of trauma).
- Reduced or abolished respiratory drive as a result of the factors that cause central nervous system depression (see above).
- Reduced respiratory effort caused by muscle weakness or nerve damage associated with conditions such as:
  - Myasthenia gravis
  - Guillain-Barré syndrome
  - Multiple sclerosis
  - Poliomyelitis
  - Motor neurone disease
  - Muscular dystrophy.

Cardiac abnormalities

These may be further classified as primary or secondary cardiac abnormalities (Resuscitation Council (UK), 2002).

Primary abnormalities include:

- Myocardial ischaemia and infarction.
- Hypertensive heart disease.
- Valve disease.
- Drugs such as tricyclic antidepressants, digoxin and anti-arrhythmics.
- Illicit drugs such as cocaine, heroin and amphetamines.
- Electrolyte imbalance.
- Hypothermia.
- Electrocution.

Secondary abnormalities that may cause cardiac arrest include:

- Asphyxia due to airway obstruction or apnoea.
- Tension pneumothorax.
- Acute blood loss.
- Severe hypoxaemia.
- Septic shock.

Causes of isolated respiratory arrest

Moulton and Yates (1999) identify four main circumstances in which isolated respiratory arrest, or failure of ventilation in the presence of a clear airway and a central pulse, may occur:

- Poisoning with narcotic agents.
- General brainstem depression associated with, for example, trauma, stroke or drugs.
- Respiratory failure.
- Neuromuscular paralysis.

How do I handle the situation?

Ultimately, whether the patient suffers an isolated respiratory arrest initially or a cardiorespiratory arrest, the emergency response follows guidelines established by the Resuscitation Council (UK) (2005b). The Council acknowledges that the level of resuscitation skills required by individual members of the healthcare team will differ according to their role in the service. This applies equally to in-hospital healthcare staff, as well as those in primary care (Resuscitation Council (UK), 2005c).

Within hospital practice, the Resuscitation Council (UK) (2005c) recommends that all healthcare professionals should be able to 'recognise cardiac arrest, call for help and start resuscitation'. They also make further recommendations that the skills of the healthcare staff should reflect the clinical environment of their practice. In other words if you work in an emergency department you should have advanced life support (ALS) skills as you are likely to be dealing with cardiac arrest patients on a regular basis, as opposed to someone working in an outpatients department who may only require basic life support skills (BLS). The Resuscitation Council (UK) (2005c) now acknowledges practitioners' levels of competence and therefore you should only perform a skill if you are competent in doing so. For example, if you are competent in the use of airway adjuncts and they are available, they should be used appropriately. Nursing staff should have been trained to a standard and level of competence compatible with their level of experience and expected duties within the hospital. Healthcare professionals who work in isolation or who may be the first responder to a cardiac arrest situation should also be trained to use an automated external defibrillator effectively.

Within the primary care setting, however, community nursing staff may find themselves as a first responder, on their own, with a collapsed patient who may have a respiratory or cardiorespiratory arrest within the home. In this situation the nurse may have to call for paramedic support and undertake BLS until the paramedics arrive. Emphasis continues to be placed on the rapid initiation of BLS as an immediate first responder intervention, until ALS equipment and staff arrive on the scene.

How do I carry out basic life support?
Martin Hopkins and Keith Todd

Sequence of interventions for adult basic life support (BLS) (Resuscitation Council (UK), 2005b)

Practice points about this sequence of actions, focusing on the use of airway adjuncts and in-hospital BLS, are provided within the sequence.

Assessing patient responsiveness
- Ensure that the location around you is safe for both you and the patient.
- Gently but firmly shake the patient's shoulders and ask loudly, 'Are you all right?'
- If there is no response to this, shout for help.

Assessing the airway
- If you cannot assess the patient fully in the position he is found in, carefully turn him on his back.
- If there is no suspicion of cervical spine injury suggested by the incident, or from any available history from a witness, open the airway using a head-tilt, chin-lift manoeuvre.
- Place a hand on the patient's forehead and gently tilt the head backwards.
- Perform a visual check of the airway. If there are any secretions visible such as blood, vomit or saliva you can remove this with the use of suction. If suction is used to clear any blood, saliva, foodstuff or gastric contents from the upper airway, this should be performed with a rigid, wide-bore catheter, such as a Yankauer sucker. The sucker should only be inserted as far as its end still being visible. This should *not* be performed if there is evidence of a solid foreign object as you may inadvertently push the object further into the airway, potentially turning a partial obstruction into a complete obstruction. If there is a solid object which is visible and can be accessed easily, forceps can be used with extreme caution to remove the object.
- At the same time, using one or two fingers on the bony point of the chin only, lift the chin to open the airway.
- You may have to loosen any tight clothing around the neck. Dentures may be left in situ if they are firmly in place; they help to maintain the shape and structure of the mouth and may make it easier to create and maintain an airtight seal around it. However, they should be carefully removed if loose, as they may become a risk to the airway.

Assessing the airway: Practice points
• Use the chin-lift manoeuvre rather than a hand placed underneath the patient's neck. The anatomy of the mouth, tongue and oropharynx means that this achieves a more patent airway and less resistance to airflow, and hence easier assessment of breathing and subsequent assisted respiration, if required
• Use one or two fingers only on the chin. Using the entire hand on and under the chin tends to impinge on the floor of the mouth and press these soft tissues up into the oropharynx, occluding the airway

Assessing breathing

Keeping the airway open, look, listen and feel for no more than 10 seconds before deciding that breathing is absent. This requires you to:

- Look for chest movements (much easier to ascertain if you place your cheek close to the patient's mouth and look towards the patient's feet, observing for rising and falling of the chest wall).
- Listen for breath sounds from the patient's mouth. These sounds should not be confused with agonal breathing (occasional gasps, laboured or noisy breathing). This is common in early stages of cardiac arrest and must not be mistaken as signs of life. Agonal breathing is present in 40% of cardiac arrest patients (Resuscitation Council (UK) 2005b).
- Feel for air upon your own cheek.

All three of these observations should take place in the same 10 seconds.

If the patient has a pulse or is showing signs of life:

- Summon help or go for help if you are on your own and call the medical emergency team using local hospital cardiac arrest call, e.g. 2222.
- Check for continued breathing on your return.

Assessing breathing: Practice point
• Appropriately trained and competent staff should be able to assess circulation by checking for the presence or absence of the carotid pulse for no more than 10 seconds at the same time as checking for breathing

- Turn the patient into the recovery position.
- Assess patient using the ABCDE approach
- Give oxygen (high flow via a non-rebreath mask if possible).
- Attach monitoring equipment if available.
- Insert intravenous cannula if skilled to do so.

If the patient is not breathing

- Send for help, if no-one has arrived already in response to your first shout, or go to summon help if you are on your own.
- Remember early defibrillation increases your patient's chances of survival.
- On your return, if you have not already done so, carefully turn the patient onto his back.
- Commence cardiopulmonary resuscitation: Give 30 chest compressions followed by two ventilations.

If any difficulty is experienced while attempting to inflate the patient's chest

- Try to tilt the head further and increase chin lift.
- Recheck that the mouth is clear of any obstruction. Remove of any secretions with suction, if available.
- Ensure that your lips are well sealed around the patient's mouth.
- Even if your rescue breaths are unsuccessful, continue with compressions until help arrives to perform advanced manoeuvres or the patient shows signs of life.

Assessing the circulation

Look for any signs of movement, including swallowing or breathing (more than the occasional gasp).

- If you have been trained to do it, check the carotid pulse. Check for no more than 10 seconds while checking breathing.
- If you are confident that you can detect signs of a circulation:
  - Give oxygen.
  - Continue to provide rescue breathing until the patient starts to breathe on his own.
  - About every 10 breaths (or about every minute), recheck for any signs of circulation, checking for no more than 10 seconds each time.
  - If the patient starts to breathe normally on his own but remains unconscious, turn him into the recovery position. You should stay with the patient and be ready to turn him on to his back once more and restart rescue breathing if he stops breathing again.

If the patient is not breathing: Practice point

- Evidence now supports chest compression before rescue ventilations as improving patients' cardiac output and therefore their oxygen circulation, increasng their chances of survival (Resuscitation Council (UK), 2005b).
- This is best carried out kneeling next to the patient or on a short step next to the bed allowing easy access directly above the patient's chest.
- If unsure of hand position, the heel of one hand can be placed in the centre of the patient's chest. Place your other hand on top and interlock your fingers. Ensure pressure is applied over the patient's sternum and not over the ribs. Correct anatomical placement of hands is the middle of the lower half of the sternum.
- The chest should be depressed 4–5cm at a rate of approx 100 times a minute or just under two compressions a second (Resuscitation Council (UK), 2005b).
- The amount of air required to ventilate a patient is difficult to estimate during basic life support, and in practice is the amount required to produce a visible lifting of the chest.
- Remember the potential dangers of over-inflation (gastric dilatation and regurgitation and aspiration of stomach contents).
- The Resuscitation Council (UK) (2005b) states that the exact timing is not critical: wait for the chest to fall completely, giving the patient approximately 10 breaths per minute.
- If in-hospital airway management and ventilation are required, this should be undertaken with the most appropriate equipment immediately available.
- Simple adjuncts such as a pocket mask, which can be used in conjunction with an oral airway, should be available in a hospital setting.
- Alternatively, a laryngeal mask airway and bag-valve apparatus, or bag-valve-mask device, can be used.
- Supplemental oxygen should be given as soon as possible (Resuscitation Council (UK), 2005c).
- Maintain the head-tilt, chin-lift position while ventilating the patient.
- Pinch the soft part of the nose and place your lips around the mouth.
- Do not forget the need to obtain a good seal around the patient's mouth, and to provide two, even, controlled rescue breaths.
- Only a small amount of resistance should be felt during mouth-to-mouth.
- Ventilation: You are observing for the chest wall to rise normally, this should take around 1 second. Allow for the chest wall to fall, and air to expire.

If there is no pulse or signs of life or you are at all unsure, start chest compressions

Locate correct position on the chest, as above, and start chest compressions:

- Position yourself directly above the patient's chest, with your arms straight, and press down on the sternum to depress it between 4 and 5cm.
- Release the pressure without allowing your hand to lose contact with the patient's chest, and repeat this at a rate of around 100 times a minute, completing 30 compressions per cycle. Allow equal time for the compression phase and the release phase, to allow the chest to return to its normal position after each one.
- Combine rescue breathing with compressions.

The Resuscitation Council (UK) (2002) recommends that, as the likelihood of BLS alone restoring effective cardiac activity is remote, time should not be wasted in further checks for the return of a pulse.

If the patient makes any sort of movement or takes a spontaneous breath, check the carotid pulse, taking no more than 10 seconds to do this. Otherwise do not interrupt cardiopulmonary resuscitation.

Continue resuscitation until:

- Qualified help, such as a medical emergency team with ALS skills and equipment, arrives and takes over.
- The patient shows signs of life.
- You become exhausted.

A final note

The sections on cardiorespiratory arrest and BLS provide an overview of your actions, essentially as a first responder in either primary or secondary care, and summarise a great deal of information and guidance available from the Resuscitation Council (UK) and other authors in the field. These guidelines are under constant review. Modifications are made to individual actions within the sequence and to the actual sequence of interventions itself as new evidence comes to light. It is essential that you keep yourself up to date with these (see www.resus.org.uk for information). Theoretical instruction and aide-mémoires such as this are no substitute for approved education and training in the skills, together with an integral assessment of competence required to practise these safely. You may find that the resuscitation training department within your own healthcare trust takes the same view, and will seek you out, on your appointment and regularly thereafter, to keep you up to date. The Resuscitation Council (UK) guidelines have removed the confusion and occasional fear previously associated with the management of cardiorespiratory arrest. If you have the opportunity subsequently to participate in the team management of one of these events, there is no better place to be than right in the centre, performing chest compressions. If you demonstrate competent and effective skills in this, no-one will bother you, other than occasionally to ask if you would like a rest. You will rarely find yourself in such an absorbing, interactive learning situation.

Chest compression: Practice points

Ensure correct hand position throughout the procedure
- Keeping your hands in contact with the chest throughout each phase of the compressions will promote this.
- Relocating the correct position, if you are performing both rescue breathing and compressions, you may find it easier to place your hands in the centre of the chest rather than locating the middle of the lower half of the sternum.

Ensure correct body posture
- Performing compressions in clinical practice can be quite tiring. Keeping your arms straight, pivoting at the hip and using your upper body weight is less tiring than trying to apply pressure using your arm muscles. Pressure should be firm, controlled, and applied vertically. You should try and change with a colleague every 2 minutes to prevent exhaustion.

Ensure correct depth of compression (4–5cm in an adult patient)
- This is difficult to estimate from a correct body posture, i.e. vertically above the patient's chest. In most cases, you will encounter a certain resistance as you approach the natural limits to the patient's chest wall 'elasticity'.
- After each cycle of 30 compressions, tilt the head and lift the chin again and give another two rescue breaths. In-hospital resuscitation with simple adjuncts may involve the use of the bag-valve-mask or laryngeal mask airway and bag-valve device. A pocket mask at the very least should be available in every clinical area. This will allow safe airway management while giving supplementary oxygen.
- Relocate the correct hand position and repeat the 30 compressions phase, continuing this cycle of compressions and breaths in a 30:2 ratio.

Ensure correct compression rate (about 100/min)
- Counting aloud '1 and 2 and …12 and 13–14–15' helps you to get into a rhythm and also provides any second person providing inflations with an audible cue.

Ensure equal compression/relaxation phases
- Patients' chests often do not rebound as readily as a training manikin. You need to allow the ventricles to refill adequately to maintain optimum cardiac output with your compressions.

Ensure correct ratio of compression:ventilation (30:2)
- This allows a more fluent resuscitation event than the previous 15:2 ratio, enhancing coronary and cerebral perfusion pressures during compressions.

Ensure interruptions to compressions
- Chest compressions should only be interrupted for rescue breaths and defibrillation
- Finally, remember that even competent, well-performed cardiac compressions will only achieve a cardiac output that is, at best, less than 30% of normal (Resuscitation Council (UK), 2002).
- Any deviation from good technique detracts from this, and further compromises the patient unnecessarily.

What are the principles of preparing patients for tests and investigations?

Penny Harrison

Duchscher (2008) suggests that the newly qualified nurse experiences a range of anxieties relating to the 'reality' of practice in the period of transition from student to registered nurse. Major foci of these anxieties include the perception of how much nurses feel they do not know. This can be applied to the knowledge relating to preparing patients for tests and investigations. However there is a wide range of help at hand. It is beyond the scope of this chapter to list every common test and investigation with its related nursing care. Rather this chapter aims to share some principles of preparing patients for a variety of tests and investigations that can be used regardless of the specialty or type of healthcare setting that nurses find themselves in. A useful resource that you can develop for yourself is your own small reference guide. I suggest that you have a hardbound notebook of A5 size, small enough to be carried in your uniform pocket. You can add information about tests and investigations related to your area of practice as you participate in caring for a number of patients. You could also use this notebook for information gained from other chapters in this book, helping to build your own unique reference guide.

Key principles of preparing patients for tests and investigations

Duchscher (2009) suggests that expectations that newly qualified nurses have about their own level of skills may reflect under-confidence and uncertainty. In my experience as a ward manager, newly qualified nurses

---

Activity break 1

Activity
- Identify the area that you are currently working in and the experienced qualified nurses that are working with you.
- Ask your colleagues if they feel confident that they have knowledge and skills relating to every test and investigation that patients may undergo.
- Ask your colleagues where they would go for further information if needed.

Reflection
- Did it surprise you that your colleagues did not necessarily know everything about every test/investigation that a patient can undergo?
- What skills did your colleagues tell you about that they utilise if they need to seek further information about tests and investigations?

Activity break 2

Activity

List the common tests that are undertaken for patients in your clinical setting. You might want to list them into groups as follows:

- Blood tests: haematology, biochemistry, microbiology, others
- Radiological tests: x-rays, computerised tomography (CT), magnetic resonance imaging (MRI), ultrasound, angiography
- Endoscopic tests: oesophagogastroduodenoscopy (OGD), sigmoidoscopy, colonoscopy
- Other tests: e.g. swallowing assessment by the speech and language therapist (SALT)

Reflection 2

Using your list as a basis for reflection, do you:

- Know what the tests/investigations are for, what information about the patient's condition will be gained?
- What care the patient requires prior to the test?
- What care the patient requires during the test?
- What care the patient requires after the test?

are often a harsher judge of their abilities than experienced colleagues who are supporting them through the period of preceptorship. The key to learning about the wide range of tests and investigations that patients undergo is to:

- Identify the common tests/investigations that take place in the current clinical setting – become familiar and confident with the 'everyday'. Do not worry about remembering the detail for every possible test and investigation.
- Know where to find further information and who you can ask for further advice/assistance; colleagues across the healthcare team prefer that you ask if unsure and are usually keen to share knowledge, expertise and experience with you.
- Participate actively in the care of the patient before, during and after the test/investigation. Seeing the patient journey through tests and investigations helps you to remember the detail of care required.
- Reflect on how much you do know and are confident with. This will help you to identify gaps in knowledge and clinical experience. Remember you can make this into an action plan for completing the preceptorship programme, as well as using this evidence as part of your ongoing professional development to meet Post-registration education and practice (PREP) requirements (Nursing and Midwifery Council, 2008b)

Patient information

Drossman (2005) defines typical questions that patients ask prior to tests and investigations:

- Why do I need this test?
- How is it carried out?
- Where do I go for this test?
- How do I prepare for this test?
- How long will it take?
- When do I hear the results?
- What do the results mean?

Patient information is not only important for the sharing of information and communication with the patient, but also as part of the process of gaining consent. Additionally, it enables the patient to cope with the test/investigation. Thus an informed patient is much better able to co-operate with the healthcare team during the test. Sufficient time spent preparing the patient for the test/investigation will be beneficial in terms of a speedy conclusion and satisfactory outcomes for both the patient and healthcare team (Bloom and Webster, 2006).

Activity break 3

Activity
- Familiarise yourself with local practice on the giving of information prior to tests and investigations.
- Ensure you know where to find patient information forms that relate to the tests and investigations that you are preparing patients for in your practice setting.

Reflection
- Reflect on how you and the healthcare team would give patients information about tests and investigations when:
  - The patient is confused
  - The patient is blind or deaf
  - The patient requires information in another language.

Consent

An important part of preparing patients for tests and investigations is gaining their consent. Nurses perform many aspects of care for patients on a daily basis, for example assisting with meeting activities of living or observations.

The Code of Conduct (Nursing and Midwifery Council, 2008a) states that the patient's consent and co-operation for care must be given. For many parts of care, verbal consent is sufficient. For example, assisting the patient to wash and dress requires the nurse to gain verbal consent from the patient, but not formal written consent. However, for more invasive tests and investigations, such as some of those identified by you in *Activity Break 2*, written consent is required.

The Department of Health (2001) has issued guidance on consent, with a set of standard consent forms introduced across the NHS in April 2002. In practice, the consent form is used in conjunction with the local consent policy. For example, local policy will usually require written consent for tests and investigations of an invasive nature, but not for less invasive procedures such as blood tests. The consent form requires the practitioner to give demographic information about the patient, list the tests/investigations or procedure to be carried out and any particular risks that the patient may be exposed to. However, emphasis is placed on the *validity* of consent, where correct completion of the consent form is the evidence of this, rather than a completed form which does not truly reflect the patient's consent to treatment or reflect true understanding about the benefits of the test, information to be gained and any potential risks or complications.

Activity break 4

Activity
- Familiarise yourself with your local trust's policy on consent.
- Ensure you know where to find the consent forms in your practice setting.
- From your lists of common tests and investigations that you identified in Activity Break 2, identify which require verbal consent and which require written consent.

Reflection
Reflect on how you and the healthcare team would gain consent for tests and investigations from:
- A patient who is confused
- A patient who has communication difficulties
- A patient who does not have English as a first language
- A patient in an emergency situation.

Pre-, peri- and post-test care

The specific pre-, peri- and post-test care for all tests and investigations is beyond the scope of this chapter. However there are some key principles that the nurse needs to be familiar with before preparing patients for tests and investigations. Alexander et al (2006), Dougherty and Lister (2008) and Walsh and Crumbie (2007) all have excellent chapters on the preparation of patients for tests and investigations, as well as details on specific care. Information from these texts can be summarised as:

- *Pre-test care*: Communication, patient assessment, information giving, consent, sedation or anaesthesia, observations, specific blood tests.
- *Peri-test care*: Communication, patient assessment, privacy and dignity, positioning and comfort, pain relief, observations, specific care.
- *Post-test care*: Communication, patient assessment, information giving, recovery from sedation (or anaesthesia), positioning and comfort, pain relief, observations, specific care.
- Follow-up care.

Activity break 5

Activity
- Familiarise yourself with the care required for a patient undergoing an oesophagogastroduodenoscopy (OGD).
- Using the checklists in the text, identify the care required for a patient undergoing an OGD in your practice setting.
- If you are not sure about the specific care involved, identify from where you would seek further advice, help and information.

Reflection
Reflect on:
- The aspects of care that you were familiar with.
- The aspects of care that you were not familiar with.
- The sources of help you could utilize.

Using the information in this chapter, reflect on how you can continue to acquire knowledge and skills to nurse patients in your practice setting for a range of tests and investigations.

Record keeping

The Nursing and Midwifery Council (2005) requires practitioners to maintain accurate, chronological records relating to all aspects of patient care. Effective record keeping is a key tool in maintaining high standards of professional practice. Record keeping for tests and investigations may involve recording information about aspects of the care and management of the patient with observations and fluid balance management as well as records of how well the test/investigation was tolerated and the recovery process. Additional information that is equally important to have recorded includes details of communications between the patient, the family or carers and the multi-professional team. Reflection of the nature of the meeting and details of how a patient received or appeared to receive information is a unique part of the role of the nurse. The records assist the nurse to co-ordinate care across the team in a co-operative and constructive manner (Nursing and Midwifery Council, 2008a). A key part of record keeping in relation to patient safety during tests and investigations is the correct labelling of specimens. Many specimens will be sent for review/reporting by technical staff within laboratories. Inaccurate labelling of specimens may delay further pathological reporting, but also has the potential to be dangerous if mixed with other patient specimens. Information relating to the patient's condition may be diagnosed incorrectly, treatment delayed or unnecessary treatment commenced. Thus safe handling of specimens is as important as other aspects of record keeping.

Activity break 6

Activity
Familiarise yourself with the care required for a patient undergoing an oesophagogastroduodenoscopy (OGD).
• Identify the patient records and charts required.
• Identify the process for labelling of specimens taken from the patient undergoing OGD in your practice setting.
Reflection
• Reflect on the wide range of records that you would use to maintain accurate patient records for this test/investigation. Did your list include any of the following ?
  • Medical notes and x-rays
  • Consent form
  • Results from blood tests
  • Admission documentation, nursing notes
  • Discharge documentation, letter to the GP
• Reflect on the range of documentation used. Was there scope for duplication or omission of information?
• Reflect on the process used to label specimens. Is there any risk of error in this process. What is the role of the nurse in minimising such risk?
• What can the nurse/nursing team do to minimise the risk of duplication/ omission?

Drug administration

The Nursing and Midwifery Council (2008b) requires practitioners to administer medications to patients in a safe manner. See questions on drug administration in *Chapter 4*.

Drugs required for tests and investigations may include sedatives prior to the test, pain relief during the test or prophylactic antibiotics to prevent or reduce the risk of infection following the test.

Activity break 7

Activity
- Familiarise yourself with the care required for a patient undergoing an oesophagogastroduodenoscopy (OGD).
- Identify the drugs required.

Reflection
- Reflect on your knowledge about the drugs used for the patient.
- Were you familiar with the drugs?
- The rational for their use?
- The potential side effects?
- Were any drugs used for a potential emergency during the OGD?

Final point

The principles underlying the administration of tests and investigations apply across all healthcare settings. The principles also fit well with the modern professional agenda for the NHS and healthcare, i.e. that of the Darzi review (Department of Health, 2008) plus the Lean (NHS Institute for Innovation and Improvement, 2007) and the Productive (NHS Institute for Innovation and Improvement, 2009) agendas. The nurse is well placed to co-ordinate care for patients requiring tests and investigations across the healthcare team (Nursing and Midwifery Council, 2008a; Duddle and Boughton, 2007). However, it is unrealistic to expect the nurse to be an expert at all tests and investigations. Competence and confidence in using these principles of management of care will assist the nurse to ensure that the patient gains the best standard of care possible while undergoing a wide range of tests and investigations.

What is a syringe driver?
Nicola Brooks

A syringe driver is a portable battery-operated infusion pump that delivers drugs via a continuous subcutaneous route at a predetermined rate (Dougherty and Lister, 2008). It should be used for patients who are unable to tolerate medication via an oral route, and has become a well-established technique for delivering analgesia, antiemetics and sedatives.

The advantages of using a syringe driver are:

- Avoids the administration of intermittent injections.
- Allows a mixture of drugs to be given together (subject to compatibility).
- Ensures accurate infusion times.
- Syringe drivers are lightweight and portable, which makes them ideal for use in the community setting or for ambulatory infusions.
- Drugs are delivered over a 12 or 24-hour period (depending on the device used).

There are very few disadvantages to using this type of device. However, the nurse must be sure which type of device is being used – a 12-hour or 24-hour device – in order to determine the correct flow rate. Before setting up an infusion device, you must be familiar with the correct operational technique. Also, the cannula and skin site need to be selected carefully, as infection and inflammation may occur.

Selection of infusion sites

Recommended sites for continuous infusion are the lateral aspects of the upper arms and thighs, the abdomen, anterior chest below the clavicle and the back (although this is only very occasionally used). A winged infusion set is used, commonly known as a 'butterfly' line. The procedure for inserting a butterfly line is as follows:

- Explain the procedure and gain the patient's consent.
- Assist the patient in adopting a comfortable position.
- Clean the chosen site with an alcohol-impregnated swab and allow to dry.
- Pinch the skin.
- Insert the needle into the skin at a 45° angle and release the pinch. Check that the needle is angled downwards into the subcutaneous tissue and not upwards into the superficial skin layer.
- Tape the butterfly 'wings' using a transparent dressing.
- Document the date and time of the procedure in the nursing notes.
- Check the patency of the line before commencing an infusion.

How do I monitor central venous pressure?
Nicola Brooks

Central venous pressure (CVP) is the pressure in the right atrium of the heart (Mooney and Comerford, 2003). It is measured by inserting a central venous catheter into the right atrium and connecting it to a manometer. The indications for monitoring a patient's CVP (Mooney and Comerford, 2003) are:

- To monitor haemodynamic status in patients who are critically ill.
- To monitor patients postoperatively.
- To facilitate the diagnosis of cardiac failure.
- To administer IV medication where the medication is an irritant when give by peripheral infusion (to monitor its effects on CVP).
- To administer large volumes of fluid (to monitor their effect on CVP in situations such as shock).
- To administer parenteral nutrition.

A 'normal' CVP reading can vary, so when you are recording a measurement it is important to ascertain at what range the medical team would like readings to be maintained. Research suggests that a simple manometer set gives a range of $3-12$cmH$_2$O, whereas with a transducer set the normal range is $0-8$mmHg. It is also important to take serial readings to establish a trend, so that abnormalities can be detected (Hatchett, 2000).

Taking a CVP measurement

With advances in medical technology, CVP measurements are now normally measured with a transducer set, particularly in critical care environments. If these facilities are not available, measurements can however be taken manually.

The CVP measurement can be taken from either the mid-axilla (so that the baseline of the manometer set is in line with the right atrium) or the sternal notch. However, it is important to take readings from one position to ensure accuracy of the result. Readings taken for the sternal notch are about 5cmH$_2$O lower than those taken from the mid-axilla.

The equipment required consists of:

- Infusion stand.
- Manometer set.
- Bag of fluid for readings (normally 0.9% sodium chloride).
- Spirit level.

Procedure for CVP measurement

- Explain the procedure to the patient and gain his/her consent.
- Gather the necessary equipment.
- Connect the manometer set to the infusion stand, and run the fluid through the infusion line. (Always seek advice if you are unsure of the procedure.)
- Use the spirit level to make sure that the patient is level with the zero marker on the manometer set to ensure an accurate result.
- Turn off the three-way tap to the patient. This will allow the manometer to fill slowly with fluid from the infusion bag. Do not overfill the chamber.
- Turn off the three-way tap to the infusion fluid. This will cause the fluid in the manometer set to fall.
- The reading can be taken when the level of fluid stops falling and settles to a rise and fall with the patient's respiration.
- Record the CVP reading on the patient's observation chart and report any abnormalities to the medical team.
- Turn off the three-way tap to the manometer and adjust the infusion rate as per prescription (to keep CVP line patent).
- Document in the nursing notes where the reading has to be taken from (mid-axilla or sternal notch) to ensure accuracy of future readings.

What do I need to know about wound dressings?
Nicola Brooks

There is a huge variety of wound dressings available, with companies competing with each other to produce the ideal dressing. Dressings are split into two categories: primary and secondary. A primary dressing is one that is in direct contact with the wound, and a secondary dressing is one that is superimposed over a primary dressing.

Factors to consider when selecting a dressing:

- Ritualistic practice. (Is it something that has always been used?)
- Evidence-based practice.
- Clinical experience.
- Resources available (expense, availability).
- Patient preference (comfort).
- Where the wound is situated.
- Size of the wound.
- What will work for which type of wound.

Characteristics of the optimum wound dressing

The ideal dressing in wound care is one that provides optimal conditions for wound healing and prevents further damage to the surrounding areas. Turner (1985) identifies several classic characteristics of the optimum dressing. Such a dressing would need to:

- Maintain a high humidity between the wound and dressing (to promote a faster rate of epithelialisation).
- Remove excess exudate and toxic compounds.
- Allow gaseous exchange.
- Provide thermal insulation at the wound surface.
- Be impermeable to wound bacteria.
- Be free from particles and wound contaminants.
- Allow removal without causing trauma at dressing change.

Types of wound dressing

The main types of wound dressing are:

- *Hydrocolloids*: These interact with wound exudate when in contact with the wound. They slowly absorb fluid to change the state of the dressing by forming a gel. This type of dressing can be used on infected wounds. The dressing should extend approximately 2cm around the wound edge.

- *Hydrogels*: Used to deslough/debride wounds. When in contact with the wound they absorb exudate to provide a moist environment. These dressings are available as a flat sheet or gel, but require a secondary dressing to keep them in place.
- *Alginates*: Manufactured from seaweed, they form a gel when in contact with a wound. Suitable for use on exudating wounds.
- *Hydrofibres*: Used to deslough/debride wounds as a primary dressing for moderate to heavily exudating wounds. Available as a woven pad or ribbon of hydrocolloid fibres.
- *Foams*: Used for exudating flat or cavity wounds with differing absorbencies. Should not be used on dry wounds because of the risk of adherence.
- *Vapour-permeable films*: These are used to treat shallow wounds, or prophylactically to prevent pressure damage, or as a retention dressing. They can be left in place for up to 7 days; however, care must be taken on removal to prevent trauma to fragile skin. The skin around the wound must be kept clean and dry.
- *Tulles*: An open-weave cotton dressing impregnated with paraffin, which requires frequent changes to prevent it drying out. It is difficult to remove if adherent, and becomes embedded in granulation tissue.
- *Iodine-based products*: These dressings contain an antiseptic, although the effects of the dressing may be reduced by the presence of pus or exudate. They can cause sensitivity in some patients.
- *Silver-based products*: These dressings have antibacterial properties contained in a dressing or cream form. Side-effects have been reported with the long-term use of silver. The dressings can be used prophylactically as a dressing on line insertion sites, e.g. Hickman lines.
- *Wound manager bags*: These products are used to control exudate on high output wounds and protect the surrounding skin. Ideally they are used to monitor the yield of exudate from a wound. They can be left in place for a long period.
- *Larval therapy*: Larvae are not often a first-line choice of wound dressing. The sterile larvae of the common greenbottle (Lucilia sericate) are used to debride the wound and remove bacteria. They are used and disposed of according to strict protocol, and ordered specifically for single patient use.
- *Vacuum-assisted closure (VAC) therapy:* VAC is used to apply negative pressure to a specialised dressing positioned in the wound cavity. Nursing staff may require extra training in the use of VAC pumps and

equipment to use them effectively. The dressing can be left in situ for a few days.

- *Paste bandages*: These products consist of cotton bandages impregnated with a medical paste. Secondary dressings are required to secure them in place. Allergic reactions are common. Paste bandages are often used in the treatment of thrombophlebitis.

When using any form of wound dressing, careful patient assessment is essential. It is advisable to use a wound assessment tool to ensure reliable and consistent documentation. Wounds should be reassessed regularly to evaluate the treatment given, as no single product is suitable for all wound types or all stages of healing. A flexible approach to the selection of wound care products is required to optimise the healing process.

What does an aseptic technique involve?
Nicola Brooks

Aseptic technique is a method of preventing micro-organisms from reaching vulnerable sites (Dougherty and Lister, 2008). An aseptic technique is used to prevent contamination of wounds that could lead to infection, and is achieved by ensuring that only sterile equipment is used during invasive procedures. The aseptic technique procedure has continually evolved from ritualistic and evidence-based practice and is a skills-based procedure (Preston, 2005).

The equipment required consists of:

- Sterile dressing pack.
- Fluid for irrigation (if required).
- Appropriate dressing.
- Hand hygiene preparation (according to local policy).
- Dressing trolley.
- Scissors.
- Tape.
- Plastic apron.

Procedure for aseptic technique

- Explain the procedure to the patient and gain his/her consent. Ensure patient comfort before the procedure.
- Clean the dressing trolley with alcoholic preparation (according to local policy).
- Place required equipment on the bottom shelf of the trolley.
- Take all equipment to the patient's bedside, and put on plastic apron.
- Loosen the dressing around the wound.
- Wash your hands and apply bactericidal alcohol hand rub.
- Check the sterility of all equipment – open the sterile field using only the corners of the paper.
- Open all other sterile packs and tip contents onto the sterile field.
- Wash your hands again and apply bactericidal alcohol hand rub.
- Place your hand in the disposable bag (inside the dressing pack) to remove the used dressing. Invert the bag and stick onto the dressing trolley.
- Put on sterile gloves, touching only the wrist end of the gloves.
- Irrigate or clean the wound as necessary.
- Change the dressing as required.
- Dispose of all used equipment in the clinical waste after the procedure.

What is involved in catheterisation and catheter care?
Penny Tremayne

Urinary catheterisation is 'the insertion of a hollow tube using an aseptic technique to enable drainage of urine or instillation of fluids as part of medical treatment' (Robinson, 2007: 48).

What measures can be taken to avoid catheterisation?

Too many individuals who are catheterised go on to develop a catheter-related urinary tract infection, so unless this invasive procedure is essential then as a nurse you have a responsibility to ensure that all possible measures are explored to avoid it. It should be a last option unless there is a medical emergency. The following are some of the options that you may wish to explore.

- Try to normalise all elimination requirements. The environment within which patients are placed may restrict their function; they may become inhibited through embarrassment or fear. Therefore, if possible, avoid the use of bedpans and commodes and encourage the patient or assist the patient in being mobilised to the toilet. Create an environment that facilitates elimination, this means a clean environment, an environment as free from disturbance as possible and somewhere where the patient is able to cleanse afterwards. If use of a bedpan/commode is unavoidable then ensure the dignity of the patient.
- If patient feels they wish to pass urine and are having difficulty perhaps because of dysuria then you may wish to consider some of the prompts that 'make you want to go', including running a tap – the splashing may trigger a wish to pass urine – or a hot bath which may cause the bladder to relax. You need to ensure that you have documented all options that you have explored.

When is catheterisation likely to be considered?

Catheterisation is likely to be considered:

- Postoperatively: to accurately monitor urine output.
- In acute illness: e.g. post-myocardial infarction or heart failure.
- For urinary retention: e.g. postoperatively or enlarged prostate gland.
- For urinary incontinence: as a last resort and only after full investigation and implementation of other management strategies.
- In the terminally ill or unconscious: to prevent possible breakdown in skin integrity.

Catheterisation exercise

Have a look at the equipment provided for catheterisation in your area. Reflect on the choice of catheters following the material, size and length criteria. Does this enable you to individualise the choice for patients past and present that you have or are catheterising? If not why not and how can you remedy this situation?

- Other indications: to determine residual urine volume; to empty the bladder before investigation; to teach intermittent self-catheterisation; and intravesical instillation of drugs (Stewart, 2001).

Catheterisation may be carried out for the following reasons:

- To empty the bladder pre-operatively or postoperatively and before specific investigations.
- To relieve urine retention.
- To determine residual urine.
- To measure accurately urine output.
- To bypass obstruction.
- To relieve incontinence (when there is no other practicable means).

If catheterisation is going to be inevitable then Bissett (2005) considers that a thorough risk assessment must be completed before the insertion. This should include patients' viewpoints, their attitude towards the insertion, which might be influenced by their age, gender, sexual activity and body image. You also have to assess patients' level of knowledge and understanding about the insertion; patients with cognitive impairments may continually pull at the catheter and cause trauma to the urethra and therefore the risks may outweigh the benefits (Bissett, 2005).

What type of catheter should be inserted?

There is a wide range of catheters available; careful assessment of the correct size and appropriate material will help to minimise complications. The main criteria for the selection of an appropriate catheter are the material it is made from, and its size and length. As a registered nurse you need to ensure that you are able to provide a rationale regarding your selection.

Material of the catheter
Consideration must be given to the length of time the catheter may be in use when selecting the material as you want to avoid unnecessary repeated

invasive interventions such as re-catheterisation. Bond and Harris (2005) and Robinson (2009) consider the following materials:

- *Polyvinyl chloride (PVC)*: This is a short-term catheter that can be used for a maximum of 7 days. It can cause discomfort if used in the long-term in that it is rigid and inflexible.
- *PVC non-balloon*: This is often used for intermittent self-catheterisation.
- *Teflon-coated with a latex core*: Because of the risk of latex allergy a majority of urinary catheters in acute area settings will be of this type. While they are regarded as short-term their recommended usage time is 28 days. Teflon coating can become thin and therefore make them unsuitable for patients with a latex allergy.
- *Silicone*: This is regarded as a long-term catheter in that it can be used for 12 weeks. If used suprapubically it can be difficult to remove as cuffing can occur.
- *Hydrogel-coated latex*: Another long-term catheter, this can be used for up to 12 weeks. This material is very compatible with body tissue and therefore can cause less trauma, but being only coated with hydrogel means it is unsuitable for those with a latex allergy.
- *Silicone elastomer-coated latex*: This catheter material helps to reduce the potential for encrustation, but, again, because it is only coated it is not suitable for those with an allergy to latex.
- *Hydrogel-coated silicone*: This is for long-term use (12 weeks) and is suitable for patients with a latex allergy.
- *Silver/silver-coated catheters*: These appear to inhibit bacterial colonisation. According to Bardsley (2009) silver has a broad spectrum activity against gram-positive and gram-negative organisms. By gradually releasing silver ions (between 10–30 days) they can reduce biofilm formation and therefore reduce bacterial adherence. They are however more costly and this has sometimes mitigated against their use. However as a nurse you need to think of long-term benefits versus short-term costs and ultimately the benefits to the patient.

The size of the catheter

All humans are all unique and that includes our dimensions, even that of our urethra. This means therefore that one size of urinary catheter does not fit all.

Catheter size is most usually measured in Charrière (Ch). This refers to the external diameter of the catheter, 1 Charrière is equivalent to 0.3mm and hence the external diameter of an 18Ch catheter is 6mm. Sometimes you may see the measurement of the catheter as Fg, meaning French gauge.

As a general rule of thumb you should always opt for the smallest catheter possible, usually 12–14Ch (Madeo and Roodhouse, 2009). However, with suprapubic catheters the size of catheter should be no smaller than a size 16Ch as this facilitates maintenance of a tract between the skin and bladder (Bond and Harris, 2005).

You need to consider past medical history and the reasoning for a catheter; if the patient has previously had a catheter inserted this may have dilated the urethra. If the person has haematuria and clots in the urine then a larger catheter will be required to drain the bladder.

What length should the catheter be?

Ever heard of the terms 'male' and 'female' catheter? These terms should be avoided but they can refer to the length of catheter available.

The female urethra is shorter than the male and therefore the catheter required for a woman will also usually be shorter, the usual length being 20–26cm. A longer catheter is used for men (up to 45cm) but a longer catheter can also be used for women who have genital oedema since the valve of a shorter catheter could cause friction and trauma. A longer catheter may afford the patient greater freedom and mobility, so the patient should be assessed carefully.

Insertion of a urinary catheter

Equipment required

- A catheter pack or dressing pack should be used, whichever provides you with the equipment you require. In some areas all-in-one Foley trays may be used which include the equipment required, including a pre-connected drainage bag (Madeo and Roodhouse, 2009).
- Sterile gloves (two pairs if required) and apron.
- Appropriate catheter – take two (one spare).
- Local anaesthetic (for both genders).
- Room-warmed normal saline (for cleaning the site).
- Syringe and sterile normal saline or water (to inflate catheter balloon, if necessary, many catheters now come with a pre-filled syringe).
- Catheter drainage bag.

Dealing with a blocked catheter

A catheter that is not draining any urine and appears to be blocked or is leaking should initially be checked for the following:

- The catheter and drainage tubing are not kinked.
- The catheter drainage bag is below bladder level.

Procedure for inserting a urinary catheter in a female patient

- Ensure consent for the procedure is elicited. Describe the procedure to the patient and the invasive nature of it, do not proceed until the patient has a clear understanding.
- Does the procedure really have to be undertaken at the bedside – if so why? Think of alternatives, it could be a treatment room where equipment is close to hand and lighting is good. Otherwise prepare the environment so it is clear of clutter and that maximum dignity can be maintained.
- Female patients are best placed in a supine position with knees bent, hips flexed and feet resting apart (they may keep covered at this stage). Older ladies may find it difficult to maintain this position, therefore an alternative position with them lying on their side could be better; this would mean that the nurse would be inserting the urethral catheter to the back of the patient. This can be quite disconcerting so another nurse should face the patient explaining the procedure.
- Wash hands, put on disposable apron.
- Prepare the trolley: open equipment packs, placing the equipment required on the top shelf.
- Wash hands. Put on two pairs of gloves. Two gloves may not be appropriate if the nurse is able to differentiate between hands that are 'clean' and 'unclean' – it is personal preference.
- Place sterile towels so the urethral orifice/meatus is exposed.
- Separate the labia minora and clean around the urethral orifice/meatus with gauze swabs, using single downward strokes. Insert the nozzle of the prescribed anaesthetic gel into the urethra and squeeze out the content (usually 3–4ml is required).
- Remove one pair of gloves if necessary.
- Insert the tip of the catheter into the urethral orifice. Advance for approximately 10–15cm until urine is detected. If the catheter has been inserted into the incorrect orifice, for example into the vagina, then do not remove it, leave it temporarily in situ and ask another nurse to place the spare sterile catheter on the sterile field. Once the catheter is correctly positioned then remove the mis-placed catheter (Robinson, 2004).
- Inflate the balloon according to the manufacturer's instructions.
- Withdraw the catheter slightly and connect to the drainage system.
- Ensure patient comfort, and that the area is clean and dry.
- Measure the amount of urine yielded.
- Dispose of all equipment in a clinical waste bag.
- Document all details relating to the procedure (catheter type and batch number, size, balloon size, date) in the nursing notes.

Procedure for inserting a urinary catheter in a male patient

- Depending where you work, male catheterisation can be perceived as an extended skill so ensure that you adhere to local policies regarding education/training requirements prior to undertaking this procedure.
- Ensure consent for the procedure is elicited. Describe the procedure to the patient and the invasive nature of it, do not proceed until the patient has a clear understanding.
- Does the procedure really have to be undertaken at the bedside – if so why? Think of alternatives, it could be a treatment room where equipment is close to hand and lighting is good. Otherwise prepare the environment so it is clear of clutter and that maximum dignity can be maintained.
- Position patients in a comfortable position as their condition dictates.
- Wash hands, put on disposable apron.
- Prepare the trolley: open equipment packs, placing the equipment required on the top shelf.
- Wash hands. Put on two pairs of gloves. Two gloves may not be appropriate if the nurse is able to differentiate between hands that are 'clean' and 'unclean' – it is personal preference.
- Wrap a swab around the penis (retracting the foreskin if necessary) and clean the glans penis with normal saline. Insert the nozzle of the prescribed anaesthetic gel into the urethra and squeeze out the content. Massage the gel along the urethra. Remove one pair of gloves if you have adopted the two glove approach.
- Grasp the shaft of the penis, raising it until it is extended. Insert the catheter slowly for approximately 20cm, until urine flows.
- Inflate the balloon according to the manufacturer's instructions. Ensure that the foreskin is un-retracted.
- Withdraw the catheter slightly and connect to the drainage system.
- Ensure patient comfort, and that the area is clean and dry.
- Measure the amount of urine yielded.
- Dispose of all equipment in a clinical waste bag.
- Document all details relating to the procedure (catheter type and batch number, size, balloon size, date) in the nursing notes.

- The catheter drainage bag is not full.
- There is no other obstruction, such as occlusion of the inlet valve by the strap of a leg bag.
- The patient is not constipated. Pressure on the drainage lumen can prevent the catheter from draining.

A common method for unblocking a catheter is a 'bladder washout'; its efficacy is debatable and the use of such terminology is confusing. At present it appears that the nurse should do what he/she can to prevent the blockage of a catheter. This includes ensuring that the patient maintains a high or at least recommended fluid intake. While this may not aid with unblocking a catheter it may prevent complications such as bladder spasms, constipation and dehydration.

- Monitor urine pH for alkalinity at least weekly or more frequently (Gates, 2000; Rew and Woodward, 2001). Burr and Nuseibeh (1997) found that catheters block more often when the urine has a high pH, so aim to keep the pH below 6.8.
- Monitor the life of the catheter for each individual patient and use one of an appropriate material.
- Change the catheter before blockage can occur.
- Optimum management of a frequently blocked catheter is to change it – check the old catheter tip for encrustations on removal.
- Inform medical staff: detrusor instability is a possibility and an anticholinergic may need to be prescribed.
- A catheter maintenance solution may be used to dissolve the minerals which may be leading to the catheter being encrusted, so it is important to note the tip of the catheter on removal.

Removing a catheter

If possible, catheters should normally be removed at night or in the early morning, so that any urine retention problems can be dealt with during the day. The equipment required to remove a catheter is as follows:

- Disposable gloves (non-sterile).
- Syringe for deflating balloon (normally 10ml).
- Clinical waste bag.
- Urine measuring jug.

The catheter balloon fails to deflate

If a catheter balloon will not deflate:

- Look for the obvious. Is there anything obstructing the catheter tubing? Is it kinked? Is there faecal impaction?
- Is there encrustation that may be dissolved by a catheter maintenance solution?

Procedure for removing a urinary catheter

- Explain the procedure to the patient and gain consent. Inform the patient of any potential problems that may occur after removal of the catheter (e.g. urgency, frequency or discomfort from irritation of the urethra by the catheter).
- Empty the residual content of urine in the drainage bag into a measuring jug and record amount on the fluid balance chart.
- Wash your hands and put on gloves.
- Use syringe to deflate the balloon. Robinson (2003) considers that removal can cause urethral trauma and highlights how 0.5ml of sterile water can smooth potential ridges and creases that can contribute to bleeding on removal.
- Ask the patient to relax, and slowly breathe in and out. On exhalation, gently and slowly remove the catheter (Robinson, 2003).
- Clean the patient, and make him/her comfortable.
- Dispose of all equipment in a clinical waste bag.

- Is the syringe that you are using faulty? Try another one.
- Leave the syringe in situ to drain spontaneously.
- Attach a needle to a 10ml syringe and insert the needle into the side arm of the catheter (above the inflation valve) and drain water gently.
- Inform medical staff if the catheter balloon still cannot be deflated (Rew and Woodward, 2001).

Final note

Catheterisation should always be a last option unless the intervention is part of emergency care delivery. Before you catheterise anyone it may be useful to think of the chain of events that, in the worse case scenario, can occur as a consequence of this invasive procedure: Patients are catheterised, they go on to develop a urinary tract infection, they develop an above normal body temperature which leads to confusion, the confusion leads to unsteadiness when mobilising and a fall; an x-ray indicates a fracture and an operative procedure follows; limited mobility causes a chest infection and the risk of other healthcare acquired infections. Ultimately death can follow. On the death certificate it will not state 'catheteristation' as the cause of death but ultimately this could be the source of that cause. So, beware, and think before catheterisation.

How can I promote continence?

Penny Tremayne

There are few things that erode a person's self-esteem and dignity more than incontinence. Many people who suffer from incontinence are often too embarrassed to seek help, even from their GP or practice nurse, and consequently suffer in silence. It is important that the nurse takes a positive approach to the promotion of continence and, if necessary, its management. Good communication and social skills are required if the nurse is to build up the essential nurse–patient relationship that is crucial in this situation.

Incontinence of urine

Incontinence of urine can de defined as the involuntary leaking of urine. It is important to recognise that there are different types of incontinence:

- *Stress urinary incontinence*: This is when there is a small amount of urine lost due to an involuntary leakage on effort or exertion or sneezing or coughing (NICE, 2006). This can be attributed to the incompetence of the urethral sphincter mechanism to close (Yates, 2008) and can occur as a consequence of constipation, being overweight and childbirth.
- *Urge urinary incontinence*: This is when a larger amount of urine is expelled (that of a full bladder) due to an involuntary leakage accompanied or preceded by urgency. According to Yates (2008) this may have no cause but can be associated with conditions where there is some neurological deficit, such as dementia, stroke, spinal injuries and diabetes.
- *Mixed urinary incontinence:* This is when there is an involuntary leakage that can be associated with urgency and exertionery factors such as sneezing and coughing (NICE, 2006).
- *Overactive bladder syndrome*: This is associated with frequency and urgency with or without urge incontinence. There may be some leakage and a desire to void more than once in the night (NICE, 2006).

NICE (2006) considers that there are three main aspects that should be considered in relation to incontinence, namely, assessment and investigation, conservative management and surgical management. Surgical management will not be considered within this section but be mindful that a referral to an appropriate surgeon may be required.

Assessment and investigation

Careful assessment is required as to the type of urinary incontinence the individual is presenting with; referral to a continence advisor may facilitate this important process. Urinalysis should be undertaken to detect blood, leucocytes, glucose, protein and nitrates in the urine. If urinalysis indicates the presence of leucocytes and nitrates then a mid-steam specimen should be obtained and, according to culture results, appropriate antibiotics prescribed.

After the individual has voided it can be useful to undertake a bladder scan to establish residual urine in the bladder. The NICE (2006) guidelines also consider the usefulness of bladder diaries that take into account the variations in usual activities; this should be maintained for a minimum of three days. There are a number of urodynamic investigations that can be undertaken to assist in assessment.

Conservative treatment

Conservative treatment is where the nurse can make a real difference with a number of health education issues that can be raised in care delivery, although this can depend on the type of incontinence. For example, caffeine reduction can be trialled for individuals with overactive bladder syndrome. Patients with a body mass index of more than 30 who have urge incontinence or an overactive bladder should be advised of the benefits of weight loss. In women with stress or mixed incontinence a three month pelvic floor training programme should be initiated. In patients who have a cognitive impairment, prompted and timed toileting programmes can be recommended. Drug treatments may be an option and these will be influenced by the type of urinary incontinence. Non-therapeutic interventions that NICE (2006) consider include absorbent products and if these are used it is essential that the appropriate product is selected, so manufacturers' instructions should be consulted. Toileting aids such as urinals may be suitable, if so, referral to occupational therapy may be required. If the urinary incontinence is long-term then more invasive measures will have to be considered, such as urethral catheterisation or suprapubic catheterisation but, with the associated complications previously acknowledged, this will have to be considered carefully.

Incontinence of faeces

One of the biggest taboos in society today can arguably be incontinence of faeces. Rees and Sharpe (2009) describe it as being one of the most embarrassing, socially unacceptable and demoralising of symptoms, and is often associated with diarrhoea, particularly in the acute care setting. All nurses need to handle this distressing symptom with great sensitivity and be aware of the NICE guidelines (2007) so they can be guided appropriately. NICE (2007) offer guidance in relation to baseline assessment, initial management, medication, specialised management, specialist assessment, long-term management, management of specific groups, and surgery. Not all of these are appropriate to discuss but a few relevant aspects should be considered.

In relation to the assessment of bowel habit a full history and examination will be required. In relation to diet, bowel opening and toilet access NICE (2007) suggests the following;

- Recommend a diet that promotes an ideal stool consistency and predictable bowel emptying – this may be aided by maintaining a food and fluid diary.
- Consider undertaking a malnutrition assessment.
- Encourage individuals to have their bowels open after eating – offer this to the individual ensuring private toilet facilities which are ideally close by and that are private and can optimise the position of sitting or squatting.
- As a nurse you may require the expertise of an occupational therapist for aids to facilitate bowel emptying as well as clothing that is easy to remove.
- An anti-diarrhoeal drug may be considered but not when the stools are hard or infrequent, or where there is acute diarrhoea without a diagnosed cause or an acute flare up of ulcerative colitis.
- Appropriate continence products must be made available and more practical advice can include planning a journey to ensure toilet access.
- A bowel management system may be considered in high dependency or palliative care settings (Rees and Sharpe, 2009) or anal plugs in those who can tolerate them (NICE, 2007).
- If incontinence persists then the individual should be referred to a specialist.
- In those who have faecal loading and this is contributing to the diarrhoea then rectal treatment may be prescribed until the bowel is cleared satisfactorily.
- In those who are prone to impaction/faecal loading then an individualised plan should be negotiated. If laxatives are used then it should be recognised that these can have side-effects and can contribute towards incontinence.

Continence clearly is very complex and Lomas (2009) highlights that while nurses are content to discuss bladder and bowel function they are deficient in specific education and training. Remember, as a registered nurse you are accountable and responsible for what you do or do not do so you may wish to consider this an aspect of care that you wish to develop professionally.

What do I need to know about pressure areas?
Penny Tremayne

Arguably, the development of a pressure ulcer within the healthcare setting can be seen as an indicator of the quality of nursing care that a patient is receiving. Costs of pressure ulcers are significant, not only financially to the NHS, but also emotionally and physically to the patient.

How do I identify whether a patient is at risk of developing a pressure ulcer?

Pressure ulcer assessments are commonly used within the clinical practice setting, although Saleh et al (2009) consider that clinical judgement may be as effective as employing a risk assessment scale to assess risk. For example have you ever undertaken a pressure ulcer risk assessment and the result indicates that the individual is not at risk yet you still think they are? In this situation, because you are professionally accountable and responsible for your actions, you should implement interventions despite the result of the assessment. The Royal College of Nursing (RCN) (2005) indicates that ulcer assessment should include the following:

- Cause of the ulcer.
- The site and location of the ulcer.
- The dimensions of the ulcer.
- Stage of the ulcer.
- Exudate – amount and type.
- Signs of local infection.
- Pain.
- Appearance of the wound.
- Appearance of the surrounding skin.
- If there is evidence of undermining or tracking – sinus/fistula.
- Odour.
- Involvement of the Tissue Viability Nurse.

This should in turn be supplemented by tracings of photography.

Which patients are most at risk of developing a pressure ulcer?

The RCN (2005) identify those individuals at increased risk of developing a pressure ulcer. These include:

- The seriously ill.
- The neurologically compromised.
- Those with impaired mobility.
- Immobility.
- Impaired nutrition.
- Obesity.
- Poor posture.
- Spinal cord injury.
- The elderly.
- Pregnant mothers.
- Infection including osteomyelitis.

What are the grades of a pressure ulcer and what do they mean ?

The European Pressure Ulcer Advisory Panel (2003) in the RCN (2005: 26–7) guideline identify the following grades:

- *Grade 1*: Non-blanchable erythema of intact skin. Discolouration of the skin, warmth, oedema and induration of hardness may also be indicators, particularly in individuals with darker skin.
- *Grade 2:* Partial thickness skin loss involving epidermis, dermis or both. The ulcer is superficial and presents clinically as an abrasion or blister.
- *Grade 3*: Full thickness skin loss involving damage to or necrosis of subcutaneous tissue that may extend down to, but not through, underlying fascia.
- *Grade 4*: Extensive destruction, tissue necrosis, or damage to muscle, bone or supporting structures with or without full thickness skin loss.

Practice points: Pressure ulcers

- Are pressure sore dressings changed according to the care plan
- What does the pressure ulcer look like?
- Is there any exudate?
- If so, is it mild, moderate or heavy?
- Is the pressure ulcer epithelialising, granulating, sloughy, necrotic, infected or fungating/malodorous?
- Compare the appearance with the photograph or original measurement template.

What care does the RCN guideline suggest regarding mobilising and re-positioning ?

The RCN (2005) indicates that care should be individualised. Mobilising should be actively encouraged and if mobilising is not an option then positioning and re-positoning should be 'frequent' and recorded. Positioning on the bony prominences, back of the head, temporal region of the skull, ear, shoulders, elbows, hip, thigh, leg, buttocks, rib cage, sacrum, knees, heels and toes should be avoided. This can also include the ischial tuberosities, parts of body affected by anti-embolic stockings (ensure correctly measured for and fitted), parts of the body where pressure, friction and shear are exerted in the course of daily activities, parts of the body where there is external force from clothing or equipment. Nasal cannulae, for example, can cause possible breakdown of skin integrity on the bridge of the nose, inside the nose, on the cheeks, and in the ear. In those who are immobile then passive limb movements should be given (RCN, 2005).

If the patient is at risk of developing a pressure ulcer, then follow the stages of the nursing process, ensure that there is a realistic, accurate and individualised care plan agreed and that this is implemented and evaluated accordingly. The care plan will include a goal – what is to be achieved. This can be immediate, but is more usually medium term or even ongoing, but must include a review/goal date. So, for example, a generic ongoing goal for a patient at risk of developing pressure ulcers might be:

Mr/Mrs/Ms/Miss .... will not develop any pressure ulcers as a consequence of being in the healthcare setting.
Review: Every Sunday

A more specific goal for a patient who has developed a pressure ulcer might read:

Mr/Mrs/Ms/Miss..................... 's Grade 3 pressure ulcer will show signs of healing and be ....mm reduced in width, ...mm reduced in length, and ....mm reduced in depth by ....[date].

The care plan should be evidence based and can include care such as that outlined below (this list is not exhaustive):

*   Adoption of an appropriate moving and handling procedure to reduce damage to the skin from shearing and friction, applying local protocol/ policy for patient handling.

- The use of pressure cushions and appropriate mattresses, the RCN (2005) in their guidance stipulate the following:
  - Grade 1–2: at a minimum high specification foam mattress or cushion with pressure reducing properties. If the ulcer deteriorates then an alternating pressure mattress of continuous low pressure system should be used.
  - Grade 3–4: the minimum provision should be an alternating air pressure mattress or continuous low pressure system. The RCN (2005) guidelines go on to clarify that the first choice of alternating air pressure mattress should be an overlay system unless there are contra-indicators such as the weight of the individual.
- Maintain or promote a balanced diet and adequate hydration – to minimise the patient's vulnerability to pressure as well as maintain elasticity of the tissues.
- Make sure that the skin is clean, dry and well moisturised. Cleanse skin as soon as possible after soiling, use mild detergents in conjunction with warm water to prevent drying and irritation, and apply moisturiser to any dry skin There are also some non-water-based foams available, which clean and moisten the skin.
- If the patient requires a dressing for a pressure ulcer, as a registered nurse you should select one that is clinically effective. The RCN (2005) consider that dressing choice should be 'modern'. Dressings should:
  - Allow excess exudate to be removed from the wound surface
  - Provide a moist micro-environment
  - Be sterile/contaminant free
  - Not shed dressing material in the wound
  - Reduce wound pain
  - Be easy to remove and apply
  - Not cause allergic reactions
  - Not cause any trauma when removed
  - Be impermeable to micro-organisms
  - Provide thermal insulation.

Evaluation

A judgement on the effectiveness of the delivery of care should be made if the patient's condition improves or deteriorates, or on the review/goal date. Thus the previous stages, such as assessment and planning, might have to be revisited.

How do I help my patients meet their nutritional needs?

Penny Tremayne

As a registered nurse, you are ultimately responsible for ensuring that patients' nutritional needs are met. At times there can be a tendency to focus on the more technical aspects of feeding, such as parenteral and enteral feeding methods.

How should I perceive mealtimes?

Mealtimes should have a high priority. It is important that patients who are acutely ill have appropriate nutritional input. Patients who are recovering perceive mealtimes as an important social event in the day, as well as providing appropriate constituents for body repair. As a registered nurse, you should try to facilitate an environment that is conducive to eating, e.g. reduce disturbances (Anderson, 2000) and try to make sure that patients have the opportunity to use a commode before mealtimes. Communicate effectively with catering, nursing and domestic staff (Horan and Coad, 2000). Make sure you act as a role model: demonstrate the importance of nutritional monitoring by getting involved, observing, and monitoring and recording whether patients are eating or being given the opportunity to eat. Some patients might not eat much because they are anxious or worried, so take the opportunity to talk to your patients and use the meal as a prompt to ask them how they feel. In some areas mealtime solutions have included a 'red ray' scheme to highlight vulnerable individuals (Davis, 2007).

How can I recognise if a patient is at risk of being malnourished?

Assessment of nutritional status is pivotal and should include the following:

- Identification of the patient's 'norm'; too often, phrases such as 'eats well' or 'no problems' are included in admission details. Explore further. What food does the patient eat? What food does he/she prefer? Is he/she physically able to shop? Can the patient afford the food or the fuel to cook the food? Is he/she physically able to cook? What amount of food does the patient normally eat?
- Assess the patient's ability on admission and on an ongoing basis. Is the patient able to eat, e.g. does he/she have dysphagia? Is the patient

able to feed him/herself? Does the patient have any specialist or therapeutic dietary needs?

- Undertake an ongoing nutritional risk assessment. The Malnutrition Universal Screening Tool (MUST) is a five-step screening tool to identify adults who are malnourished or at risk of malnutrition. The five steps of MUST are (British Association for Parenteral and Enteral Nutrition, 2008):
  - Measure the height and weight of the individual to calculate body mass index (BMI).
  - Note the percentage of unplanned weight loss and score appropriately.
  - Establish acute disease effect and score appropriately.
  - Add the scores from the three previous steps and an overall risk of malnutrition will be obtained.
  - Use management guidelines and/or local policy to develop care plan.
- Weigh the individual as appropriate.
- Observe the individual's general condition and bodily appearance and document accordingly.

What can I do if a patient is not eating very much?

If the patient is not eating very much:

- Try to identify the cause. Is it related to a sore mouth, coated tongue, nausea, vomiting, abdominal discomfort, constipation, diarrhoea or pain?
- Encourage the family to bring in food that the patient likes and to actively participate in the nutritional care of the individual, but only if this is appropriate.
- Maintain an accurate fluid balance and food chart. Avoid writing phrases such as, 'fish – all'. What does this mean? There is difference between a whole cod and a sardine. Specify the amount eaten, whether it is a teaspoonful or a tablespoonful.
- Offer nutritional supplements as appropriate and as prescribed.
- For other supplements and dietary advice, request appropriate referral and/or prescription. Some supplements can potentially be harmful as they have high levels of nutrients (Barton et al, 2000; Green, 2000). Patients unable to be adequately nourished by mouth may receive enteral feeding via a nasogastric tube (often fine bore) or percutaneous endoscopic gastrostomy.

Procedure for inserting a nasogastric tube

- Explain the procedure to the patient and gain consent.
- Take all the equipment to the bedside and ensure patient privacy.
- Wash hands and put on gloves.
- Ensure that the patient is sitting comfortably – ideally sitting upright.
- Estimate the length of tube to be passed by measuring the distance from the nose to the earlobe, and down to the xiphisternum. Use your second hand to hold the correct position, or use the markers on the nasogastric tube as guidance.
- Select the best nostril to insert the tube into (not tender, no deviated septum, etc.). Ask the patient to blow his/her nose or sniff through each nostril to establish the most patent nostril.
- Encourage the patient to relax and to breathe normally.
- Lubricate the tip of the nasogastric tube with water to make passing it easier.
- Pass the tube gently into the nostril, and pass backwards to the nasopharynx (if you experience difficulty in passing the tube, remove it and try the other nostril).
- Check patient comfort and allow patient to recover for a few minutes.
- Ask the patient to breathe through the mouth and swallow. At the point of swallowing, gently advance the tube into the stomach to the required length. (A sip of water given when passing the tube may assist swallowing.)
- Check the position of the tube in the stomach by one of the following methods:
  - Aspirate stomach contents with a 20ml syringe. Check to see that the pH is less than 4.0
  - Insert 5–10ml of air into the tube while another nurse listens to the stomach with a stethoscope. As air enters the stomach, a gurgling sound will be heard (this technique is not used in children). Auscultation is not reliable, and should not be used as the sole method of confirming the tube position (Methany et al, 1990).
  - X-ray to check the position (this is not necessary with a Ryles tube; however, fine-bore feeding tubes have a guidewire in place, which will show on X-ray). This is identified as best practice to check the placement of the tube, however it may delay feeding, so it is important to check the current practice within your area.
- Secure the tube in position with tape.

What are the principles of caring for patients with wound drains?

Nicola Brooks

Wound drains are widely used within the surgical setting for two main reasons:

- Removal of fluid (e.g. exudate, pus, blood and other body fluids).
- To remove air from a cavity or dead tissue space (Pudner, 2005).

The insertion of a drain provides a channel to the body surface for fluid which might otherwise collect in the wound space. This can reduce the risk of infection, and allows closer apposition of the tissues aiding the healing process (Torrance and Serginson, 2007)

There are a variety of wound drains available, but they all work by one of two mechanisms: passive drainage, using gravity to release the fluid into a collecting bag or dressing (e.g. corrugated drains, tube drains); or active drainage, using a vacuum or suction mechanism to remove the fluid.

Wound drains are used for three main reasons:

- *Therapeutic drainage:* This is used to remove infected material such as bacteria, pus or dead tissue from the body, or to reduce the dead space within a wound to prevent abscess formation. Surgical techniques used for therapeutic drainage include needle aspiration, incision and drainage, and complete surgical excision.
- *Prophylactic drainage*: This is used to prevent infection, but it has been replaced by the use of antibiotic therapy and has now largely been abandoned.
- *Decompressive drainage:* This is intended to prevent leakage of urine, bile, intestinal and pancreatic fluid, or to prevent fluid accumulating either within or around the wound, to reduce the risk of further complications.

Complications of wound drains

There are relatively few complications associated with wound drains. However, Torrance and Serginson (2007) have identified some risks:

- The drain is a 'foreign body', which may impair healing.
- Inflammation.
- Movement or misplacement of the drain.
- Kinking or obstruction of the tubing.

- Breakage or accidental removal.
- Pain.
- Tissue in-growth.
- Fluid and electrolyte loss.

Nursing management of drains

Observation and careful handling of wound drains are of paramount importance within the practice setting. There are many factors that should be taken into account when caring for a patient with a drain in situ. An aseptic technique should be used when handling the drainage system, which should be disturbed as little as possible to reduce the risk of infection (Pudner, 2005).

Monitoring the drain/drainage fluid
The colour, amount, and nature of the drainage fluid should be recorded onto the fluid balance/wound drainage chart. Excessive drainage or changes in the type of fluid (particularly fresh blood) should be recorded and reported to the medical team.

Observation of the drain/drain site
Observe the drain site for damage to the surrounding skin caused by inflammation or fluid exudate. Gloves should be used when handling drains or the drainage system. Check that the drain system is well secured with no kinks or obstruction of the tubing that may hinder the drainage process. Check that the suture(s) are secure and not pulling the skin.

Dressing the site
A sterile keyhole dressing should cover the site to absorb any leakage. A passive drain should have either a sterile absorbent dressing placed over it, or a drainage bag to collect fluid. Standard precautions need to be applied when dealing with body fluid.

Patient information
Ensure that the patient is kept fully informed of why the drain is there and how long it will need to remain in place, in order to reduce anxiety, as well as provide practical assistance on teaching the patient how to cope with a drain. To ensure compliance, factors such as ensuring that the drain remains patent, effective and aseptic, and how the drain will be removed, should be explained to the patient. Patients who are mobile may be uncomfortable with the image that the drain portrays. This is particularly important in women having surgery for breast cancer. In these circumstances it may be possible to 'disguise' the drain bag as a small handbag.

Removing a drain

The drain should be removed when either the drainage has stopped; of if there is a risk of complication (e.g. infection or obstruction). Some drains are removed as standard practice after an identified period of time; however this is normally advised by medical colleagues.

Changing a vacuum drainage system bottle

It may be necessary to change the drainage bottle if the drain is yielding large amounts, or if there is a loss of vacuum to the drainage system.

Procedure for removing a drain

- Explain the procedure fully to the patient and ask him/her to get into a comfortable position before removal.
- Check the medical notes to ensure that the drain is to be removed.
- If the drain is on an active drainage system (the vacuumed/suction method), de-vacuum the drain to reduce trauma to the tissues as the drain is pulled out.
- Wash hands and apply sterile gloves. Maintain an aseptic technique during the procedure (see section on aseptic technique, p. 49).
- Cut the retaining suture.
- Gently and smoothly remove the drain (difficulty in removing the drain may indicate adhesions, so always seek medical advice if you are unsure).
- Apply a sterile dressing to the drain site, and observe for bleeding/leakage.
- Dispose of all equipment appropriately (drains are clinical waste).
- Document the procedure in the nursing notes.

Procedure for changing a vacuum drainage system bottle

- Explain the procedure fully to the patient.
- Wash hands, put on sterile gloves.
- Clamp drainage tubing near to drainage site and bottle.
- Disconnect bottle and wipe with an alcohol-impregnated swab to ensure that it is an aseptic procedure.
- Connect new bottle to the tubing.
- Unclamp both clamps.
- Ensure that the drain is patent and drainage fluid is coming down the tube.
- Remember to document drainage fluid measurements on the fluid balance or wound drainage chart.

How do I look after a nasogastric or gastric tube?
Nicola Brooks and Penny Tremayne

Nasogastric tubes are used for four main reasons:

- *Before or following abdominal surgery*: To ensure that the stomach is empty, and to relieve any anastomosis (artificial connection of internal structures) or pressure.
- *Persistent vomiting*: To reduce the risk of aspiration and ensure patient comfort.
- *Intestinal obstruction*: To empty the stomach and to ensure patient comfort.
- *Short- or long-term feeding*: For individuals who are not able to meet their nutritional requirements but have a functioning gastrointestinal tract. A fine bore feeding tube, made of polyurethane, is preferable to a PVC Ryles tube, as patient comfort is enhanced (Pudner, 2005).

Inserting a nasogastric tube

The equipment required for inserting a nasogastric tube consists of:

- Nasogastric tube of appropriate size and type, e.g. Ryles tube, fine-bore tube (fine-bore tubes are only used for feeding purposes).
- Water to assist placement of the tube.
- PH paper to check the position of the nasogastric tube.
- Receiver/vomit bowl.
- 20ml syringe.
- Clinical waste bag, tissues, tape to secure tube in position.
- Spigot or drainage bag as necessary.
- Non-sterile gloves.

Potential problems following insertion of a nasogastric tube

- *No aspirate*: If no aspirate occurs, ensure that the tube is in the correct position by checking the back of the throat for coiling. If the tube is coiled, try to re-position it slightly and re-aspirate.
- *Tube misplacement*: This is often indicated by respiratory distress or coughing. If the patient is showing signs of respiratory distress, this probably indicates that the nasogastric tube has entered the respiratory passage, and the tube should be removed immediately.
- *Unable to pass tube past nasal cavity*: Ask the patient for suggestions

as to why the tube may not pass, e.g. previous nasal surgery, injury. Try the other nostril. If you are still unable to pass the tube, then leave alone.

How do I know if the nasogastric tube is in the correct position?

Make sure you check your local policy/protocol for any specific details. Gastric aspirate on pH-sensitive paper strips should confirm the position of the tube.

- pH 3–4 indicates gastric position.
- pH >6 indicates bronchial positioning. The patient may also become distressed by coughing or gagging and appear cyanosed.
- pH 6–8 indicates that the tube has passed through the stomach into the intestine (aspirate will be green/yellow, indicating the presence of bile). Note also whether the patient is receiving medication (e.g. antacids, proton pump inhibitors) that can cause changes in the gastric pH (Burnham, 2000). If in any doubt at all, then do not commence feeding until position has been confirmed by x-ray.

What should I be specifically looking for when nursing a patient with a gastrostomy?

- Check your local policy/protocol for specific details.
- Check the site of the gastrostomy for redness, inflammation or pain.
- A dressing should only be in place for the initial 24 hours (Howell, 2002).
- Check that the tube can be rotated 360° to prevent scar tissue formation (Howell, 2002).
- If there is pain, bleeding, signs of perforation, aspiration or that the gastrostomy has been pulled out, seek medical and specialist nurse assistance immediately.

What can I do to prevent the nasogastric/gastrostomy tube becoming blocked?

- Flush the tube with water regularly, before and after every feed and before and after each drug administration (Colagiovanni, 2000; Bryson, 2001).
- Use a polyurethane nasogastric tube (Colagiovanni, 2000).

Can I administer drugs via a nasogastric/gastrostomy tube?

- Apply local policy/protocol.
- Yes you can, but you should always seek the advice of the pharmacist as there are factors that can affect drug interaction, drug dosage and method of delivery, which you need to consider (Bryson, 2001).

What should I do if the tube is blocked?

- Make sure that you check the local policy/protocol for specific details.
- Flush tube with warm sterile water.
- Milk the tube with fingers to aid 'unclogging' of the tube. There is some debate regarding the use of carbonated drinks and pancreatic enzymes, but the evidence supporting this is inconclusive, and in this instance you should be advised by medical or specialist nursing staff.

What is the nursing management of intravenous therapy?

Nicola Brooks

If a patient is unable to tolerate enough oral fluids to maintain a sufficient fluid balance, intravenous (IV) therapy will be required. This may be given on either a short-term basis, e.g. postoperatively until oral intake is resumed, or for several days if the patient is being kept nil by mouth. The most common reasons for using IV therapy are:

- Dehydration.
- Vomiting and/or diarrhoea.
- Excessive insensible loss (e.g. sweating).
- Preoperative and postoperative hydration.
- Hypercatabolism.
- Unconsciousness.

Nursing management of an IV infusion

The basic principles of caring for an IV infusion are:

- Wash hands and maintain aseptic conditions when dealing with the infusion.
- Maintain a closed system.
- Ensure that the packaging for the fluid to be infused is not damaged, and the fluid's 'use by date' is still current.
- Ensure that fluids hang no longer than 24 hours (4 hours for blood) as some solutions deteriorate in bright sunlight.
- Ensure that the cannula site is clean and dry, and checked on a regular basis for signs of infection, and that the cannula is held securely to the patient.
- It is recommended that a cannula should be re-sited after 72 hours (RCN, 2005) but this may have clinical indications depending upon the patient condition, and the availability of alternative cannula sites.
- Infusion sets should be changed every 48–72 hours (RCN, 2005). They should be changed immediately after a blood transfusion, intravenous feed or at 24 hours (whichever is sooner). For clear fluids, change after 72 hours (RCN, 2005). It is good practice to record the date and time that the set is due to be changed.
- Ensure that infusion rates are maintained accurately.
- Record and monitor an accurate fluid balance.

In order to avoid complications with the administration of IV infusions, it is important that the correct site, cannula size and infusion device are used. The appropriate size of cannula to be inserted depends on such factors as the volume and type of fluid to be infused, the duration of IV therapy, the ease of access and the patency of veins. It is also important to check which arm the patient would like the cannula sited in, wherever possible, as this may increase compliance. The non-dominant arm is recommended, although this may be contraindicated by patient condition or disease. For a cannula that is to be inserted within the wrist or antecubital fossa, a splint may be required for support and to prevent flexion.

A wealth of infusion sets is available, but the set commonly used in the clinical setting contains a valve mechanism designed to prevent air entry if the infusion fluid runs out. These also have a macro-drip system, which takes approximately 15–20 drops for every one millilitre (ml) of fluid. The number of drops per ml is variable depending on the viscosity of the fluid: approximately 15 drops for blood and high viscosity fluids, and approximately 20 drops for clear fluids.

Where smaller volumes of fluid are to be infused, or a more precise rate of flow control is required, the use of a volumetric infusion control pump device is recommended (Medical Devices Agency, 2003). Blood and blood products are given via blood administration sets, which are discarded either immediately after completion of the transfusion, after 12 hours of first use, or if the filter becomes blocked, but this may vary according to local policy.

Calculating flow control

It is important to ensure that the type of fluid, the volume, infusion time, date and signature of the prescriber are documented on the fluid prescription sheet. It is the nurse's responsibility to calculate the flow rate and ensure that the correct rate is maintained. A formula is used to calculate the correct flow rate. However, it is essential to know the number of drops per millilitre (ml) being delivered by the infusion set. (Standard infusion sets normally give approximately 15–20 drops/ml of fluid infused.)

The calculation is therefore: number of millilitres to be infused divided by the number of hours over which the infusion is to be delivered multiplied by the number of drops per ml divided by 60 minutes.

Example
A 1000ml bag of fluid to be delivered over 8 hours, using a standard infusion set (delivering 20 drops/ml), would work out as:

No. of ml to be infused	x	No. of drops per ml	=	Number of drops to be
No. of hrs infusion to run		60 mins		delivered each minute

$$(1000 \div 8) \ \times \ (20 \div 60) = 42 \text{ drops per minute}$$

Remember

Certain factors affect the flow rate, so the infusion needs to be checked regularly to ensure that it is running continuously. There should be no alterations to 'catch up' the infusion regimen. Factors affecting flow rate are:

- Cannula position, movement or patency.
- Problems with the infusion equipment, e.g. blocked filters, kinked tubing, height of fluid container.
- Infusion fluid factors, e.g. viscosity, temperature, specific gravity.
- Complications of venous spasm, e.g. infiltration, phlebitis, thrombophlebitis.

Complications of infusion therapy

- *Infiltration and extravasation*: This occurs when the infusion fluid leaks into the tissues as a result of the cannula or needle becoming displaced. There may be oedema at the site, the patient may complain of pain and the skin around the site may feel cooler than the surrounding skin. Lastly, you may feel a resistance when trying to inject fluid into the cannula. If the fluid or additive is a vesicant, then this can cause tissue necrosis, and immediate medical attention needs to be sought.
- *Infection at the insertion site – phlebitis and thrombophlebitis*: Inflammation of the vein is termed phlebitis; thrombophlebitis occurs when inflammation is further complicated by the formation of a blood clot within the vein. Phlebitis and thrombophlebitis may be caused by movement of the cannula within the vein, or by contaminated equipment or fluids. Both phlebitis and thrombophlebitis can be minimised by attention to technique and good infection control measures.

References

Alexander M, Fawcett J, Runciman P (Eds) (2006) *Nursing Practice: Hospital & Home – The Adult* (3rd edn). Churchill Livingstone, Edinburgh

Anderson P (2000) Tickling patients' taste buds. *Nursing Times* 96(50): 24–6

Armitage M, Eddleston J, Stokes T and Guideline Development Group (2007) Recognising and responding to acute illness in adults in hospital: Summary of NICE guidance. *British Medical Journal* 335: 258–9

Bardsley A (2009) Coated catheters: Teviewing the literature. *Journal of Community Nursing* 23(2): 15–16

Barton A, Kay S, White G (2000) Managing people on sip feeds in the community. *British Journal of Community Nursing* 5(11): 541–7

Bissett L (2005) Reducing the risk of catheter-related urinary tract infection. *Nursing Times Supplement* 101(12): 64–7

Bloom S, Webster G (2006) *Oxford Handbook of Gastroenterology and Hepatology*. Oxford Medical Publications, Oxford

Bond P, Harris C (2005) Best practice in urinary catheterisation and catheter care. *Nursing Times Supplement* 101(8): 54–8

British Association for Parenteral and Enteral Nutrition (2008) *Malnutrition Universal Screening Tool* , BAPEN, Worcestershire

Bryson E (2001) Drug administration via a nasogastric tube. *Nursing Times* 97(16): 51

Burnham P (2000) A guide to nasogastric tube insertion. *Nursing Times* 96(8 Suppl): 6–7

Burr RG, Nuseibeh IM (1997) Urinary catheter blockage depends on urine pH, calcium and rate of flow. *Spinal Cord* 35(8): 521–5

Colagiovanni L (2000) Preventing and clearing blocked feeding tubes. *Nursing Times* 96(17 Suppl): 3–4

Davis C (2007) Mealtime solutions. *Nursing Standard* 21(41): 21–3

Department of Health (2001) *Reference Guide to Consent for Examination or Treatment*. Department of Health, London

Department of Health (2008) *High Quality Care for All: NHS Next Stage Review final report*. (Lord Darzi's review). The Stationary Office, London

Dougherty L, Lister S (Eds) (2008) *The Royal Marsden Hospital Manual of Clinical Nursing Procedures*. Student Edition (7th edn). Wiley Blackwell. London

Drossman D (ed) (2005) *Handbook of procedures* (4th edn). Philadelphia: Lippincott Williams and Wilkins

Duchscher J (2008) A process of becoming: The stages of new nursing graduate professional role transition. *Journal of Continuing Education in Nursing* 39(10): 441–50

Duchscher J (2009) Transition shock: The initial stage of role adaptation for newly graduated Registered Nurses. *Journal of Advanced Nursing.* 65(5): 1103–13

Duddle M, Boughton M (2007) Intraprofessional relations in nursing. *Journal of*

Advanced Nursing **59**(1): 29–37

Gates A (2000) The benefits of irrigation in catheter care. *Professional Nurse* 16(1): 835–8

Goldhill D, McNarry A (2004) Physiological abnormalities in early warning scores are related to mortality in adult inpatients. *British Journal of Anaesthesia* **92**(6): 882–4

Green S (2000) Oral dietary supplements. *Journal of Community Nursing* **14**(3): 26–8

Hatchett R (2000) Central venous pressure measurements. *Nursing Times* 96(15): 49–50

Horan D, Coad J (2000) Can nurses improve patient feeding? *Nursing Times* **96**(50): 33–4

Howell M (2002) Do nurses know enough about percutaneous endoscopic gastrostomy? *Nursing Times* **98**(17): 40–2

Jevon P (2002) *Advanced Cardiac Life Support: A practical guide*. Butterworth-Heinemann, Oxford

Lomas C (2009) Nurses must receive sufficient continence education and training. *Nursing Times* **105**(21): 32–3

Madeo M, Roodhouse AJ (2009) Reducing the risks associated with urinary catheters. *Nursing Standard* **23**(29) :47–55

McBride J, Knight D, Piper J, Smith G (2005) Long-term effect of introducing an early warning score on respiratory rate charting on general wards. *Resuscitation* **65**: 41–4

Medical Devices Agency (2003) *Infusion Systems Device Bulletin*. Medical Devices Agency, London.

Methany M, McSweeney M, Wehrle,MA, Wiersema L (1990) Effectiveness of the auscultatory method in predicting feeding tube location. *Nursing Research* **39**(5): 262–7

Mooney G, Comerford D (2003) What you need to know about central venous lines. *Nursing Times* **99**(10): 28–9

Moulton C, Yates D (1999) *Lecture Notes on Emergency Medicine* (2nd edn. p 175). Blackwell Science, Oxford

NHS Institute for Innovation and Improvement (2007) *Going Lean in the NHS*. www.institute.nhs.uk/lean [accessed 1.7.2009]

NHS Institute for Innovation and Improvement (2009) *The Productive Series*. www.institute.nhs.uk/productive [accessed 1.7.2009]

NICE (2006) *Urinary Incontinence: The management of urinary incontinence in women*. NICE, London

NICE (2007) *Faecal incontinence: The management of faecal incontinence in adults Clinical Guideline 49*. NICE London

Nolan J, Deakin C, Soar J, Bottiger B, Smith G (2005) European Resuscitation Council Guidelines for Resuscitation 2005 Section 4. *Advanced Life Support Resuscitation* 67S1 S39-S86

Nursing and Midwifery Council (2002) *Supporting Nurses and Midwives through Lifelong Learning*. Nursing and Midwifery Council, London

Nursing and Midwifery Council (2003) *Professional Conduct FAQs*. http://www. Nursing and Midwifery Council-uk.org/Nursing and Midwifery Council/main/ advice/professionalConductFaqs.html [accessed 20.2.2005]

Nursing and Midwifery Council (2004) *Guidelines for the Administration of Medicines*. Nursing and Midwifery Council, London

Nursing and Midwifery Council (2005) *Guidelines for Records and Record Keeping*. London: Nursing and Midwifery Council.

Nursing and Midwifery Council (2008a) *The Code: Standards of Conduct, Performance and Ethics for Nurses and Midwives*. Nursing and Midwifery Council, London

Nursing and Midwifery Council (2008b) *The PREP Handbook*. London: Nursing and Midwifery Council.

Preston RM (2005) Aseptic technique: Evidence-based approach for patients safety. *British Journal of Nursing* **14**(10): 540–2

Pudner R (ed) (2005) *Nursing the Surgical Patient* (2nd edn). Elsevier. London

Rees J, Sharpe A (2009) The use of bowel management systems in the high dependency setting. *British Journal of Nursing* **18**(7) S19–24

Resuscitation Council (UK) (2002) *Immediate Life Support Manual*. Resuscitation Council London

Resuscitation Council (UK) (2005a) *Introduction: Resuscitation Guidelines*. Resuscitation Council, London

Resuscitation Council (UK) (2005b) *Adult Basic Life Support: Resuscitation Guidelines*. Resuscitation Council, London

Resuscitation Council (UK) (2005c) *In-Hospital Resucitation: Resuscitation Guidelines*. Resuscitation Council, London

Rew M, Woodward S (2001) Troubleshooting common problems associated with long-term urinary catheters. In: Pope Cruickshank J, Woodward S. *Management of Continence and Urinary Catheter Care*. BJN Monograph. Quay Books, Dinton, Wiltshire

Robinson J (2003) Deflation of a Foley catheter balloon. *Nursing Standard* **17**(27): 33–8

Robinson J (2004) A practical approach to catheter-associated problems. *Nursing Standard* **18**(31): 38–42

Robinson J (2007) Female urethral catheterisation. *Nursing Standard* **22**(8): 48–56

Royal College of Nursing (2005) *The management of pressure ulcers in primary and secondary care: A Clinical Practice Guideline*. RCN/NICE, London

Saleh M, Anthony D, Parboteeah S (2009) The impact of pressure ulcer risk assessment on patient outcomes among hospitalised patients. *Journal of Clinical Nursing* **18**: 1923–9

Stewart E (2001) Urinary catheters: Selection, maintenance and nursing care. In: Pope Cruickshank J, Woodward S (eds) *Management of Continence and Urinary Catheter Care*. BJN Monograph. Quay Books, Dinton, Wiltshire

Subbe C, Kruger M, Rutherford P, Gemmel L (2001) Validation of a modified early warning score in medical admissions. *Quarterly Journal of Medicine* **94**: 521–6

Torrance C, Serginson E (2007) *Surgical Nursing* (13th edn). Bailliere Tindall, London

Walsh. M, Crumbie A (eds) (2007) *Watson's Clinical Nursing and Related Sciences* (7th edn). Bailliere Tindall, London

Yates A. (2008) Identifying and managing urinary continence problems. *Practice Nurse* **36**(9): 31–6

Notes

CHAPTER 3

Dealing with grief, bereavement and palliative care

- How do I talk with patients, relatives and carers?
- How do I contact relatives/carers following a death?
- What if I am involved in caring for a terminally ill child?
- How do I care for the patient's body after death?
- How do I manage pain in palliative care?
- What are the causes of pain in advanced cancer?
- What is the analgesic three-step ladder?
- How do I manage nausea and vomiting in palliative care?
- How do I manage intestinal obstruction in palliative care?
- How do I manage constipation in palliative care?
- How do I manage dyspnoea in palliative care?
- How do I manage mouth problems in palliative care?
- How do I manage the psychological care of terminally ill patients?

How do I talk with patients, relatives and carers?
Martyn Geary

How a person responds when given news of a diagnosis or prognosis will vary enormously. It will be affected by age, gender, religion, cultural and social background and the major life experiences through which the person has lived. In addition, how people respond when given a diagnosis may echo, to some extent, how they have responded to and coped with previous major life events (Buckman, 1992; Higgins, 2002). It may be, for example, that patients or their carers have always dealt with any form of stress or crisis by pushing it to the back of their mind, trying, as far as possible, to ignore the problem and continue with their day-to-day life as if nothing untoward had happened. If this has been the person's major coping strategy in the past, it is not improbable that he/she may demonstrate similar coping mechanisms when confronted with the news of a life-threatening condition.

Authors and researchers such as Kubler-Ross (1970) have addressed explicitly the issue of patients' coping strategies and emotional responses when confronted with 'bad news'. Kubler-Ross emphasises that people's emotions and responses very often change over time; sometimes these emotions may appear contradictory – denial and unrealistic hope for the future one day, and apparently resigned acceptance of the 'inevitable' the next – as people fluctuate between different responses. The variation and changing nature of response is seen to be a perfectly normal and natural reaction to one of the most difficult situations any one of us will ever have to confront – news of a life-threatening condition. While the positive insights of Kubler-Ross' work are still as relevant today as they were 30 years ago, there are problems relating to how the insights she offers are used in clinical practice and applied by practitioners to patient care.

Writers such as Fulton and Metress (1995) argue that there is a tendency for practitioners to interpret literally stage theories, such as those developed by Kubler-Ross, and to presume that all people will pass through similar stages of 'denial', 'bargaining', 'anger' and 'depression', to arrive at the ultimate endpoint of 'acceptance'. The danger here is that practitioners may view the coping strategy displayed by individuals as one of many that they may potentially display over the course of a disease journey. While this may be true for some people, it may not be the case for others. This assumption could lead the practitioner to challenge a perceived 'unhelpful' response in the belief that, once challenged, it may be replaced by one they perceive to be more positively adaptive. Some people may have other coping mechanisms upon which they can draw, but for others it may mean that the only coping mechanism they have ever used is threatened. If it is taken from them, what are they to replace it with?

To avoid this situation occurring, it is perhaps helpful to view the work of authors such as Kubler-Ross as a model or guide to the overall complexities of emotional response displayed by individuals confronted with bad news, rather than see it in prescriptive terms – 'this is how people will behave'. The key, as always, is to listen to the patient or carer and to make an individualised assessment of the coping strategies and emotional responses displayed, and to plan interventions based on that assessment.

How do I contact relatives/carers following a death?
Martyn Geary

Informing relatives that a loved one has died is an understandably stressful situation for all practitioners, whatever their level of experience. The following guidelines may be helpful.

Before the death

- Record the name and contact telephone number of a person to be contacted in the event of a patient's deterioration. Do not assume that this will be the same as the next of kin. Consider recording two names to ensure that the name of an additional contact is known should the first be unavailable.
- Record the person's full name, not simply their surname – there may be people in the same house with the same surname.
- Clarify when this person might not wish to be contacted. For example, do they wish to be contacted during the night? If not, ascertain the time after which they do not wish to be contacted and if there is anyone else who should be contacted in their place.

Contacting relatives/carers over the telephone

- Collect all of the relevant documentation together.
- Find a private and quiet place (preferably an office or room separate from the rest of the ward or unit) where you can make the telephone call.
- Inform colleagues of what you are about to do so that you will not be disturbed.
- Check and double check that you are about to contact the right relative or carer about the right patient – mistakes can and do happen.
- Before you dial the number, mentally rehearse what you are going to say.
- When the phone is answered, introduce yourself and ask to speak to the person concerned.
- Clarify that you are speaking to the right person. Instead of saying 'Is that Mrs Smith', say instead something along the lines of 'Is that Mrs Pat Smith, Jack's wife?'
- The phone call itself will cause alarm so do not delay in giving the news. Try to convey the information slowly and sensitively without the use of euphemisms. For example, after having established that you are speaking to the right person, you might say: 'Mrs Smith, I'm afraid I've got some bad news. There's no easy way to say this. I'm sorry to say Mr Smith has died.'

- Be prepared for a range of possible responses.
- If the person wishes to come into the hospital, ensure that you make it clear how to gain access, particularly at night if the usual entrances are closed.
- Ask if the person is fit to drive.
- Ask if you could telephone anyone on their behalf.
- If they are not intending to leave for the hospital immediately, explain that you will phone back in half an hour to check on them.
- If they choose not to come in during the night, explain what needs to be done the following day.

Preparing for relatives'/carers' arrival

- Ensure that all staff members are aware of the patient's death and that relatives/carers are expected.
- If at all possible, try to ensure that a member of staff is allocated to the care of relatives.
- If relatives/carers are expected to arrive during the night, arrange for hospital security or portering staff to meet them at the hospital entrance and show them to the ward.
- Ensure that the allocated staff member is waiting for them on the ward and is there to escort them to a prepared office or quiet room. Ensure that there are sufficient chairs available and tissues at hand in the room. If there is a phone in the office, divert calls to a different extension. A busy ward office is not the ideal place.
- Ensure that the nurse allocated to the patient's care is appraised of the circumstances surrounding the death – relatives/carers are likely to have questions about what happened and the order of events. Documenting the details of events surrounding a death can also be of value if the ward or unit operates a bereavement support programme where relatives may meet with practitioners in the months following the death. Unless recorded, events around a death can be forgotten by health professionals, especially if they were not directly involved in care delivery at the time.

Being with relatives/carers

- Be sensitive to the range of possible reactions people may display.
- Remember that there is likely to be little or nothing a practitioner can say that will ease the pain that people experience. Attempting to 'reassure' can, albeit unintentionally, be interpreted as talking in platitudes.
- Recognise and accommodate religious and cultural diversity in the way that people express their grief.

- Take your lead from the bereaved. Even if people have arrived at the hospital, check that they still wish to view the body. If so, explain beforehand what they will see when they enter the bed area or side-room. Some people may never have seen a dead body and be apprehensive as to what to expect.
- Accompany carers/relatives to the bedside.
- Check with relatives if they wish to spend time alone. Providing chairs at the bedside gives them reassurance that they will not be rushed.
- How people wish to act when with the deceased will vary. Religious and cultural factors as well as personality and the effect of grief itself will influence what people wish to say or do.
- Offer access to a religious/community leader or minister if appropriate.
- Offer the opportunity for relatives/carers to speak to a member of the medical staff to discuss events surrounding the death.
- Some people may wish to kiss, hold or lie with the deceased; others may choose not to, while some may be reticent and appreciate the nurse taking the lead in touching and 'speaking' to the person who has died.
- While providing time for relatives to be alone if they wish, check regularly whether there is anything they need. Remember to point out the location of toilets and telephone facilities and offer refreshments.
- Before they leave the ward, ensure that they are given information (reinforced with written details) as to what to do and where to go to collect the death certificate and any property of the deceased. A list of support organisations should also be given.
- Ensure that all details of the visit are entered in the nursing notes.

What if I am unable to contact the person over the telephone?

In addition to trying the number at a later time, check to see if there is an alternative contact number. If no telephone number is recorded, check with directory enquiries. Failing that, you may have to consider contacting the patient's GP, if appropriate, to request a visit to the deceased's relatives, or contact the police service who can arrange for officers to visit the address to convey the information personally. There will be a procedure for contacting the police – check this with your senior nurse manager.

What if there is an answering machine attached to the telephone?

As soon as you realise that an answering machine is attached to the phone, replace the receiver without leaving a message. This will give you time to compose yourself and to rehearse what it is you wish to say. Obviously, in the message you leave, you will not tell the relative/carer about the death, but ask them to contact the ward as soon as possible, giving the name of the person with whom they should ask to speak.

What if the person collapses with the shock of the news?

Stay calm and continue speaking to the person. If they have collapsed, it is likely they will rally within a few seconds. If this does not happen and they fail to respond, check in the notes of the deceased to see whether there is an alternative contact. If not, you may have to contact the police service to ask for officers to visit the person's address to check on their welfare.

What if I am involved in caring for a terminally ill child?

Zoe Wilkes

Family-centred care

One of the major approaches when caring for a very sick child is the promotion of family-centred care. It is not only the needs of the child but also those of the whole family that have to be addressed, including those of any siblings. There is often a multidisciplinary team involved in the care of terminally ill children, providing all aspects of medical, nursing and psychological care to the family. It is important to work as a team and to coordinate and share all the treatment and care that the child and family receive. It is recognised that supporting a family during this time can be very stressful for the staff involved and it is often the nurse who plays a key role in helping the family and child prepare emotionally for the child's forthcoming death (Costello and Trinder-Brook, 2000). Brykczynska (1992) recognises that the nurse has a pivotal role in providing information and continuity of care and has the ability to empathise on a level of sensitivity and common human understanding.

Symptom control

In a publication written for staff working in a children's hospice, Jassal (2001) advises staff to listen to the parents' views and ideas regarding symptom control, as they have become the experts in their child's care. Through a focused listening process, the level of intervention and symptom control will nearly always be established.

The symptoms listed below could be exhibited at some time in some children and should form the basis of any holistic assessment (Jassal, 2001).

Common symptoms in terminally ill children	
• Anorexia	• Cough
• Infections	• Pain
• Bladder problems	• Diarrhoea
• Mouth care	• Psychological problems
• Bleeding problems	• Dyspnoea
• Muscle spasms	• Skin problems
• Constipation	• Gastro-oesophageal reflux
• Nausea	• Vomiting
• Convulsions	• Noisy breathing

The assessment should be initiated as a baseline measure, and then the child should be reassessed in an ongoing manner, depending on his/her needs.

The treatment of many of these symptoms can be of a non-pharmacological nature, e.g. changing a child's position, altering a feeding regimen, nursing in a quiet environment. However, there will be situations where relief may only be obtained through medication. In these instances it is very important to listen to the needs and choices of the family and to work closely with the appropriate medical staff in relaying this information. It is vital that the family is given the opportunity to make informed decisions and to work in partnership with the multidisciplinary team caring for the child.

Time and emotions

It is very important to organise the environment in which the child is cared for in a way that allows time, freedom and privacy for the child and carers to express their emotions in a way that they can be sensitively cared for. This will vary depending on whether the child is in an acute hospital, a hospice or is being cared for at home. Providing emotional support includes making sure that all staff are supported and have the opportunity to talk through their feelings as they care for the child and family. There is no right or wrong way to behave or feel in these circumstances. It is the responsibility of professionals to acknowledge their feelings in order to practise effectively. In most cases the family will look to the nurse involved in their child's care for support and guidance, therefore it is just as important that nurses concerned seek their own support from a source that they too feel is safe and appropriate.

How do I care for the patient's body after death?
Martyn Geary

General points

- Ensure that the death has been verified. This can be carried out by a doctor or suitably qualified senior nurse (Cooke, 2000).
- Be sensitive to the religious or cultural beliefs and wishes of patients and their community. If at all possible, these should have been ascertained and recorded within the patient's notes before the death.
- Establish whether relatives/carers wish to view the body before or after last offices have been performed. In some instances this may mean that the care of the body is undertaken by family members or community leaders, or that the nurse assists as they take the lead in the last offices.
- Be familiar with your hospital/trust policy on the removal of tubes, drains and catheters as this can vary. All should be left in place, including existing dressings, if the:
  - death is unexpected
  - death occurs within 24 hours of admission or surgery
  - death is accidental or occurred in suspicious circumstances
  - cause of death is unknown
  - patient has been brought in dead
  - death may be the result of an industrial disease.
- In all the above situations it is likely that the death will be referred to the coroner (Cooke, 2000).
- Universal infection control precautions should be adopted at all times. Make arrangements with the hospital mortuary for a cadaver bag to be available if the body is leaking body fluids or known to be infected with hepatitis B, C, human immunodeficiency virus (HIV) or other communicable infection. Minimal handling of the body is recommended in such instances to minimise the risk of contamination.
- Inform other patients of the death and provide support and reassurance as necessary.
- Be aware of the needs of colleagues, particularly those who may have been directly involved in the patient's care or those with limited experience in caring for the dying and bereaved.

Undertaking last offices

- Lay the patient's body on his/her back and straighten the limbs. Place a single pillow under the head with a rolled towel on the upper chest to support the jaw.

- Use moistened cotton wool pads and light pressure for 30 seconds to close the eyelids.
- Cover any leaking wounds with waterproof dressings. If orifices are leaking excessively, packing with gauze may be required. Drain the bladder with pressure over the lower abdomen.
- As long as it is not contraindicated by religious or cultural beliefs or by the wishes of relatives/carers, wash the body and dress it in either a shroud or personal clothing.
- Mouthcare and care of dentures should also be undertaken. If the person usually wore dentures, these should usually be reinserted in the mouth. The person's previous preferences should be respected in relation to the combing and arrangement of hair and facial shaving.
- Follow hospital/trust policy in relation to the labelling of the body. The usual procedure is to attach identification labels to one of the patient's ankles and to one of the wrists. A notification of death card is usually attached to the patient's chest before the body is wrapped in a mortuary sheet (Mallett and Dougherty, 2000).
- When wrapping the body the nurse should ensure that all limbs are secured and that face and head are covered. The sheet should be secured with tape and placed, if necessary, within a cadaver bag.
- A second notification of death card is then secured to the mortuary sheet or cadaver bag over the patient's chest.
- If relatives/carers wish certain pieces of jewellery to be removed from the body, this should be done in the presence of another nurse and be recorded on the patient's property form. If any jewellery remains on the person's body, this should be recorded on the notification of death cards (Mallett and Dougherty, 2000).
- Complete the appropriate nursing notes and arrange for the transfer of the body to the mortuary. Ensure that the patient's property is transferred (in the absence of relatives/carers) to the appropriate administrative department.

How do I manage pain in palliative care?
Wendy Taylor

What is pain?

Pain is not a simple sensation, but a complex physiological and emotional experience.

(Regnaud, 2004)

Pain is whatever the experiencing person says it is, existing whenever he says it does.

(McCaffery, 1968)

In palliative care, the effective management of pain requires:

- Thorough assessment.
- A consideration of the patient's ideas, beliefs, concerns and expectations.
- Negotiation of the management plan with the patient at all stages.
- A multidisciplinary perspective.
- A holistic approach, incorporating physical, psychological, social and spiritual aspects.
- Use of drugs, physical and psychological treatments, complementary therapies and spiritual support.

The concept of 'total pain' encompasses social, spiritual and emotional components, as well as physical, as illustrated in the box on page 96.

Pain assessment

This should be carefully and thoroughly carried out. The following should be ascertained:

- The site of the pain and any radiation (use body diagram).
- A description of the type of pain, i.e. stabbing, burning, colicky.
- The severity of the pain (scoring system can be used).
- What makes the pain better and worse.
- The effectiveness of any analgesia administered and the duration of that effect.

The concept of total pain

Physical influences
- Symptoms or debility
- Pathology
- Side-effects of treatment
- Cancer/non-cancer

Social influences
- Friends who do not visit
- Financial worries
- Loss of social position
- Loss of job prestige and income
- Loss of role in family
- Isolation

Emotional influences
- Anger:
  - Delays in diagnosis
  - Unavailable doctors
  - Treatment failure
- Fear:
  - Pain
  - Death
  - Hospitalisation
  - Loss of dignity
  - Loss of choice/control
  - Uncertainty about the future
  - Disfigurement

Spiritual influences
- Why has this happened to me?
- Death seen as punishment
- Helplessness
- Loss of self-worth
- Why does God allow me to suffer like this?
- Is there any meaning to life?
- Can I be forgiven for the past?

What are the causes of pain in advanced cancer?
Wendy Taylor

Points to remember

- Not all cancer patients experience pain.
- Not every pain is due to the cancer.
- Understanding, empathy, diversion and feeling cared for are important adjuncts to analgesia.
- Attention to detail is vital – always be asking: 'Why is this happening?'

Causes of pain in advanced cancer

- The cancer itself
  - Visceral from involvement of abdominal, pelvic or intrathoracic organs
  - Soft tissue infiltration
  - Bone involvement
  - Neuropathic
- Treatment related, for example,
  - chemotherapy-related mucositis
- Cancer-related debility, for example,
  - constipation
  - muscle spasm/tension
  - pressure sore
- A concurrent disorder, for example,
  - osteoarthritis
  - migraine
  - post-stroke pain

(adapted from Twycross and Wilcock, 2001)

What is the analgesic three-step ladder?
Wendy Taylor

The 'analgesic ladder' (*Figure 3.1*) provides a guidance framework for the administration of analgesic drugs.

How to use the ladder

- Start at the bottom.
- Work up in a stepwise progression.
- Use the maximum dose of a drug before moving up.
- Never move sideways in the same efficacy drug group.
- Titrate the drug dose upwards until the patient is pain free.
- Give analgesics by mouth whenever possible.
- Give analgesics regularly to prevent pain returning.
- Have realistic goals. Aim for progressive pain relief:
  - at night
  - at rest during the day
  - on movement (not always completely possible).
- Reassess constantly and adjust drugs/doses accordingly.
- Ensure that all patients have extra analgesia prescribed for transitory pain exacerbations.

(Twycross and Wilcock, 2001)

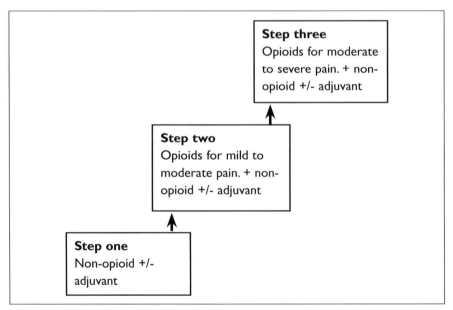

Figure 3.1. The analgesic ladder (World Health Organisation, 1996).

Drugs used on the analgesic ladder

Non-opioids
- Paracetamol.
- Non-steroidal anti-inflammatory drugs (NSAIDs).

Opioids
- Weak: codeine.
- Strong: morphine – oral strong opioid of choice.
  diamorphine – parenteral strong opioid of choice.
- Useful alternatives to strong opioids in cases of intolerable effects with morphine are:
  - hydromorphone
  - oxycodone
  - fentanyl – used in the form of transdermal patches.
- Methadone: strong opioid (but requires careful monitoring – usually commenced in a specialist unit). Useful in patients with:
  - adverse effects with morphine
  - escalating pain despite increasing doses of morphine
  - resistant neuropathic cancer pain
  - renal failure.

Adjuvants
- Antidepressants.
- Anticonvulsants.
- Steroids.
- Skeletal muscle relaxants.
- Antispasmodics.
- Bisphosphonates.
- Ketamine.

Other ways of managing pain in palliative care

- Radiotherapy.
- Hormone therapy.
- Chemotherapy.
- Surgery.
- Psychological, e.g. counselling or cognitive-behavioural therapy.
- Interruption of pain pathways:
  - local anaesthesia
  - nerve blocks
  - neurosurgery

- heat pads
- transcutaneous nerve stimulation (TENS).
- Complementary therapies:
  - acupuncture
  - relaxation
  - visualisation
  - hypnotherapy
  - reflexology
  - homoeopathy
  - aromatherapy
  - massage.

(adapted from Twycross and Wilcock, 2001)

How do I manage nausea and vomiting in palliative care?
Wendy Taylor

There are many reasons why nausea and vomiting may occur, which can make it difficult to achieve complete control.

The mechanism of vomiting

The vomiting centre is situated in the brainstem and controls and coordinates vomiting. It responds to stimuli from:

The chemoreceptor trigger zone – situated in the area postrema in the fourth ventricle. Stimulated by:
- Blood toxins.
- Biochemical abnormalities, e.g. hypercalcaemia, uraemia.
- Drugs, e.g. NSAIDs, opioids.

Area neurotransmitters – serotonin and dopamine.

The vestibular nerve – stimulated by:
- Middle ear disease.
- Motion sickness.

Area neurotransmitters – acetylcholine and histamine.

The cerebral cortex – stimulated by:
- Anxiety.
- Thoughts.
- Tastes and smells.
- Anticipation of past remembered stimulus, e.g. chemotherapy.

Area neurotransmitters – acetylcholine and histamine.

The vagus nerve – stimulated by:
- Gastric stasis.
- Constipation.
- Gastrointestinal obstruction.
- Gastric distension.
- Stretched liver capsule.
- Cough/excessive sputum.

Area neurotransmitters – acetylcholine and serotonin.

Direct stimulation:
- Radiotherapy.
- Raised intracranial pressure.

Management of nausea and vomiting

Ask why the patient is vomiting and identify possible causes. The treatment will depend on the cause. Treat potentially reversible causes (Twycross, 2002), such as:

- Constipation.
- Coughing.
- Raised intracranial pressure.
- Hypercalcaemia (if appropriate).
- Gastric irritant drugs.

Use the most appropriate anti-emetic to treat the cause (see box below).

How should anti-emetics be administered?

The route of anti-emetic administration is important. Only use oral anti-emetics for the prevention or treatment of mild nausea. For the adequate control of nausea and vomiting, anti-emetics need to be given by:

- Suppository: cyclizine, domperidone.
- Subcutaneously: either as a bolus injection, or using a syringe driver, with one or more anti-emetics: cyclizine, metoclopramide, levomepromazine, haloperidol, hyoscine. Once control has been achieved, oral drugs may be substituted (Kaye, 1992).

**Anti-emetics for use in palliative care
(Adapted from Geary, 2000)**

- Remember: One-third of patients with nausea and vomiting need more than one anti-emetic for satisfactory control (Twycross, 2002).
- Use combinations of drugs, which have different actions.
- Anxiety exacerbates nausea and vomiting irrespective of the cause.
- Consider using non-drug methods:
  - distraction
  - relaxation
  - acupuncture
  - hypnotherapy.
- Give drugs subcutaneously, not intramuscularly (less painful).
- Give an anti-emetic regularly.

Drug affinity to neurotransmitter sites and actions

Metoclopramide: Dopamine and serotonin antagonist
- Increases gastric motility
- Useful for gastric stasis

Levomepromazine: Dopamine and serotonin antagonist and antihistamine
- Useful for persistent nausea and vomiting of unknown cause
- Sedative in higher doses

Ondansetron: Serotonin antagonist
- Useful for chemotherapy-induced nausea and vomiting
- Very constipating

Lorazepam: Useful in nausea and vomiting induced by fear, anxiety

Diazepam: Anticipation of stimuli

Haloperidol: Dopamine antagonist
- Useful in chemically induced nausea and vomiting (drugs, biochemical abnormalities, toxicity)

Cyclizine: Antihistamine
- Useful in vestibular disturbances and radiotherapy to the head and neck
- Very useful if you do not know the cause of the vomiting

Hyoscine: Anticholinergic
- Depresses vomiting centre
- Dries secretions
- Antispasmodic

Corticosteroids: Useful in enlarged liver and cerebral oedema, and gastric outflow obstruction

Domperidone: Dopamine antagonist
- Useful alternative to metoclopramide
- Acts on gut wall
- Does not cross blood–brain barrier, so few central effects

How do I manage intestinal obstruction in palliative care?

Wendy Taylor

Obstruction of the gastrointestinal tract can occur at any site, from the oesophagus to the large bowel. It can be partial or complete, and acute or chronic. It can be caused by a number of factors (Twycross and Wilcock, 2001):

- The cancer itself.
- Consequences of past treatment, e.g. adhesions.
- Drugs, e.g. opioids.
- Debility, e.g. faecal impaction.
- Unrelated benign conditions.

  Symptoms of intestinal obstruction:

- Abdominal pain (colic is common).
- Vomiting.
- Abdominal distension.
- Absolute constipation (if obstruction is complete).

Management

Surgery must be considered; however, many patients are unsuitable and unfit for operation.

Nasogastric suction and intravenous (IV) fluids are usually inappropriate in prolonged inoperable obstruction.

Medical treatment

Aim to control the symptoms and allow eating and drinking (Kaye, 1992).

- Trial of high-dose steroids may resolve the obstruction (give subcutaneously), e.g. dexamethasone.
- Nausea – use cyclizine, haloperidol or levomepromazine.
- Intestinal colic:
  - stop stimulant laxatives
  - stop anti-emetics that increase gastric motility (metoclopramide, domperidone)
  - use an antispasmodic, e.g. hyoscine butylbromide
  - consider using diamorphine.

(Rudd, 2002)

A subcutaneous syringe driver can be used with a combination of drugs infused over 24 hours, e.g. diamorphine, hyoscine butylbromide, cyclizine and octreotide. Octreotide reduces intestinal secretions in bowel obstruction, thus alleviating distension and reducing the chance of vomiting and colic.

How do I manage constipation in palliative care?
Wendy Taylor

Constipation means hard or infrequent motions (Kaye, 1992). This is a common problem in palliative care patients – ask every patient about it.

Predisposing factors

- Poor diet and/or inadequate fluid intake.
- Drugs, especially opioids, also diuretics, anticholinergics.
- Immobility.
- Gut cancers.
- Spinal cord compression.
- Other diseases (e.g. diverticular disease).

Constipation can cause

- Nausea and vomiting.
- Impaction of faeces with overflow, causing spurious diarrhoea.
- Abdominal pain.
- Urinary incontinence or urinary retention.

(Rudd, 2002)

Treatment

- If possible, reverse the cause.
- Always prescribe a laxative with an opioid.
- Laxative choice: use a softener plus a stimulant, e.g:
  - Senna and lactulose
  - Senna and docusate.
- Sodium picosulfate elixir (Laxoberal for resistant cases).
- Rectal intervention:
  - Suppositories: bisacodyl (stimulant); glycerine (softener)
  - Enemas: phosphate.

How do I manage dyspnoea in palliative care?
Wendy Taylor

Dyspnoea means a distressing difficulty in breathing (Kaye, 1992). There is often more than one cause.

Common causes of dyspnoea in palliative care include:

- Anxiety.
- Lung cancer (primary or secondary):
  - obstruction of the bronchus
  - effusion.
- Anaemia.
- Other lung disease.
- Loss of respiratory muscles.
- Pulmonary embolus.

(Faull and Woof, 2002)

Remember:

- Careful assessment is required to establish the cause.
- Reverse the reversible (i.e. effusion, chest infection).
- Use drug and non-drug treatments.

Dyspnoea: Points of management

Non-drug treatment
- Explore anxieties – dyspnoea can cause panic and fear; these in turn can exacerbate the symptom. Patients often fear suffocation
- Explain the mechanism of dyspnoea
- Teach breathing exercises, relaxation and distraction technique
- Adapt lifestyle; adjust to loss of role and abilities
- Use electric fan
- Position for maximal breathing
- Listen to, support and reassure the patient

Drug treatment
- Opioids, e.g. morphine
- Oxygen if hypoxic and there are no contraindications
- Nebulised saline if there is tenacious sputum
- Bronchodilators if there is reversible airways obstruction
- For excessive, noisy secretions – 'death rattle' – use glycopyrronium bromide or hyoscine hydrobromide. Both are powerful anticholinergics; the latter is very sedating

---

How do I manage mouth problems in palliative care?

Wendy Taylor

Mouth problems in palliative care are common and can be distressing. Meticulous mouth care is vital. Dentures should be removed and cleaned thoroughly daily.

Dry mouth

This is usually the result of a decrease in the amount of saliva secreted, or a change in the composition of the saliva. The most common cause is drug therapy. Treatment:

- Saliva substitutes:
  - Oralbalance gel
  - Saliva Orthana spray
- Saliva stimulants:
  - Chewing gum
  - Pilocarpine, or
  - Bethanecol chloride (fewer side-effects than pilocarpine)

Oral thrush

Oral candidosis (thrush) can present in different forms. Features are relatively non-specific, e.g. white patches on the oral mucosa or red areas. The oesophagus can be involved, causing pain and difficulty with swallowing. Treatment:

- Antifungal drugs, e.g. fluconazole and nystatin.

If the patient does not respond to treatment, send an oral swab to microbiology.

How do I manage the psychological care of terminally ill patients?
Wendy Taylor

To contemplate understanding how a patient who is facing death feels may seem an almost impossible task. But some emotions and fears are common experiences, and there are aspects of life that are considered important by most of us:

- Work.
- Finance.
- Leisure and fun.
- Relationships and family.
- Prior experience of illness.
- Roles and status.
- Meaning of life and faith.

> *It is how each patient views and copes with each of these components when facing the end of their life that drives their emotions and subsequent behaviour.*

(Faull and Woof, 2002)

Patients who are terminally ill, facing death, can experience a psychological response similar to that which occurs in bereavement. Kubler-Ross (1970) describes five stages of dying. People may experience these stages in sequence, or may oscillate backwards and forwards between the stages:

- *Denial*: The refusal to believe the truth of what is happening.
- *Anger*: 'Why me?' This can be directed at anyone, e.g. doctor, family or friends.
- *Bargaining*: The patient tries to make a deal with someone, e.g. God, doctor, relative. 'If you cure me, God, I promise that I'll try to be a much better person.'
- *Depression*: The impending loss of life causes hopelessness, despair and anxiety.
- *Acceptance*: The patient has emotionally adjusted to what is happening. The struggle and fighting is over. Not all patients reach this stage.

Common fears of terminally ill patients include:

- The process of dying.

- Pain and other symptoms.
- Loss of control over one's body.
- Loss of control in decision making about care.
- Separation from loved ones.
- Rejection.
- The unknown.
- Dying alone.
- 'Ceasing to be'.
- Death itself.
- Letting God down.
- Unfinished business.
- Dignity.
- Altered body image.

Remember sharing fears will reduce them – ask patients what they are frightened of.

How can I help patients deal with their fears?

Dying patients should always be told the 'appropriate' truth about their diagnosis; only then will they build up trusting relationships with their professional carers, and feel safe to express their fears. However, it is important for patients to retain some hope. Most patients want to talk about their diagnosis, dying and other fears.

Fostering hope

There are several key strategies to facilitating hope (Herth, 1990):

- The presence of a meaningful relationship.
- The ability to feel lighthearted.
- Personal attributes of determination, courage, and serenity.
- Clear aims.
- Spiritual beliefs.

References

Brykczynska G (1992) Caring – a dying art. In: Jolley M, Brykczynska G (Eds) *Nursing Care: The Challenge to Change*. Edward Arnold, Kent

Buckman R (1992) *How to Break Bad News: A guide for healthcare professionals*. Macmillan, London

Cooke H (2000) *When Someone Dies: A practical guide to holistic care at the end of life*. Butterworth-Heinemann, Oxford

Costello J, Trinder-Brook A (2000) Children's nurses' experience of caring for dying children in hospital. *Paediatric Nursing* **12**: 6

Faull R, Woof R (2002) *Palliative Care*. Oxford University Press, Oxford

Fulton GB, Metress EK (1995) *Perspectives on Death and Dying*. Jones and Bartlett Publishers, Boston, US

Geary M (2000) PHCP 2052/3052: *Symptom control in palliative and terminal care*. (Unpublished paper). De Montfort University, Leicester

Herth K (1990) Fostering hope in terminally ill people. *Journal of Advanced Nursing* **15**: 1520–9

Higgins D (2002) Breaking bad news in cancer care. *Professional Nurse* **17**(10): 609

Jassal S (2001) *Basic symptom control in paediatric palliative care*. Unpublished guidelines (3rd edn). The Rainbows Children's Hospice, Loughborough, Leicestershire

Kaye P (1992) *A to Z of Hospice and Palliative Medicine*. EPL Publications, Northampton

Kubler-Ross E (1970) *On Death and Dying: Care of the patient, relatives/carers following a death*. Tavistock/Routledge, London

Mallett J, Dougherty L (Eds) (2000) *The Royal Marsden Hospital Manual of Clinical Nursing Procedures* (5th edn). Blackwell Science, Oxford

McCaffery M (1968) *Nursing Practice Theories Related to Cognition, Bodily Pain, and Man-Environment Interactions*. University of California at Los Angeles Students' Store

Regnaud C (2004) Dysphagia, dyspepsia and hiccup. In: Doyle D et al (eds) *Oxford Textbook of Palliative Medicine* (pp 468–83). New York: Oxford University Press, New York

Rudd N (2002) *A Guide to Prescribing for Patients with Advanced Malignancy*. Leicestershire Cancer Centre, Leicester

Twycross R (2002) *Introducing Palliative Care* (4th edn). Radcliffe Medical Press, Abingdon

Twycross R, Wilcock A (2001) *Symptom Management in Advanced Cancer*. Radcliffe Medical Press, Abingdon

World Health Organization (1996) *Cancer Pain Relief: With a guide to opioid availability*. WHO, Geneva

Notes

CHAPTER 4

The principles of patient medication

- What is the nurse's role in drug administration?
- What legislation governs medications and are there other national documents that guide us in this practice?
- How do drugs work?
- What are the principles of safe practice for giving medication?
- What do I need to know about drug calculations?
- What are the routes of drug administration?
- What are the ethical issues in drug administration?
- How can I avoid drug errors?
- What are the alternative and new initiatives in drug administration?

What is the nurse's role in drug administration?
Annie Law

The most frequent clinical intervention that registered nurses perform in the NHS today is drug administration. This area of practice is also the most frequent cause of anxiety in newly registered nurses. The complexity of drug regimens has increased with the continuous stream of new and novel drugs and patients receiving multiple drug therapy. This in turn increases the risk of adverse reactions and errors (Cavell, 2000). To ensure safe and effective drug administration you need to maintain your knowledge of drugs at a high level and constantly update that knowledge. This chapter aims to provide you with the minimum knowledge you need in order to be a safe practitioner in drug administration. It is not the intention to cover all the common medications as there are sufficient sources available in all clinical areas for reference purposes.

To be able to administer drugs safely, a nurse needs to have sufficient knowledge in the following areas:

- Legislation related to drug therapy.
- Pharmacology.
- Principles of safe practice.
- Drug calculations.
- Routes of drug administration.

- Ethical issues in drug administration.
- Management of drug errors.
- Alternative and new initiatives: self-administration; patient group directions; nurse prescribing.

What legislation governs medications and are there other national documents that guide us in this practice?

Annie Law

Legal and professional frameworks

Two key pieces of legislation govern the use of drugs:

- The Medicines Act 1968.
- The Misuse of Drugs Act 1971.

Although these are somewhat dated, there have been statutory instruments (secondary legislation) to supplement these Acts as changes occur.

Medicines Act 1968

This Act controls the manufacture and distribution of medicines, i.e. who can lawfully supply and be in possession of medicines, and how medicines are packaged and labelled. The Act classifies drugs into three categories:

- Prescription-only medicines (POM): Drugs that may only be supplied and administered to a patient on the instruction of an appropriate practitioner.
- Pharmacy-only medicines: Drugs that can be purchased from a chemist shop only if the sale is supervised by a pharmacist.
- General sales list: Drugs that do not need a prescription or supervision of a pharmacist – basically anything you can buy in a supermarket.

Misuse of Drugs Act 1971

This replaced the previous Dangerous Drugs Act, and controls the import, export, production, supply and possession of drugs of abuse. Changes in the legal status of some drugs have led to the Misuse of Drugs (Safe Custody) Regulations 1973 and the Misuse of Drugs Regulations 1985. These identify five separate schedules of controlled drugs, which you need to be familiar with as your responsibilities in terms of storage, checking and disposal relate to the different schedules.

Nursing implications

Any discrepancies in the stock balance of controlled drugs may result in the police becoming involved. It is therefore vital that you familiarise yourself with local policies related to controlled drugs. You must know:

- The correct storage of these drugs.
- The scrupulous checking required when administering these drugs to a patient, and the stock balance each day.
- The disposal mechanisms.
- Record keeping.

Nurse Prescribing Act 1992

This piece of legislation reached the statute books directly as a result of the need for the law to catch up with the demands of the NHS (Shepherd, 2002b); this has been further developed by Nurse Independent Prescribing (Department of Health/National Practitioner Programme, 2006).

NMC Standards for Medicines Management

The Nursing and Midwifery Council's (NMC) Standards for Medicines Management (NMC, 2008) were produced by the professional regulatory body for nurses and midwives to set standards for safe practice in the management and administration of medicines. They will be discussed in more depth later in this chapter.

European Union (EU) directive

The EU directive 92/27/EEC places a responsibility on each member of the EU to provide patients with information leaflets for each medicine dispensed. This became law in 1999.

Nursing implications
If you are teaching patients how to take their medication before leaving hospital or in their own homes, patient information leaflets provide a useful information source for you and your patient. You should ensure that the patient or carer is aware of this information, which they can refer to if necessary when you are not there.

National Institute for Health and Clinical Excellence (NICE)

NICE was set up by the Government in 1999, and although its role is to advise on best practice related to diagnostic techniques, medical devices, therapeutic interventions, as well as drug prescribing practices, its agenda has been dominated by the last category.

Nursing implications

You should keep yourself up to date with any new guidelines that NICE produce related to the prescribing of drugs for particular conditions. These guidelines can be found on the website for NICE at www.nice.org.uk.

National Service Frameworks

These frameworks have been produced by expert groups working with the Government to provide guidance to clinicians and health service managers on best practice in terms of service provision, e.g. cancer, heart disease, mental health and older people. They contain guidance on specific drug therapy.

Nursing implications

Maintaining your knowledge of any frameworks connected with your specialty will not only help you to understand any recommendations for particular drugs, but also to understand why services may change and the impact that these changes may have on nursing. The National Service Frameworks can be viewed and downloaded from the Department of Health website www.dh.gov.uk/Home/fs/en.

Other Government documents

The Department of Health published a report in 2000 entitled *An Organisation with a Memory* (Department of Health, 2000a). This report made two recommendations specific to medicines:

- To decrease to zero the number of patients dying or being paralysed by maladministered spinal injections.
- To cut by 40% the number of serious errors in the use of prescribed drugs by 2004.

The Department of Health recently published guidance for extension of the list of medical conditions giving exemption from NHS prescription charges (Department of Health, 2009). It is important that you know who can apply for exemption from prescription charges to enable you to advise your patients appropriately. People over the age of 60 are exempt on age grounds and this new guidance gives people with a diagnosis of cancer the right to apply for exemption. The same right for people with other long-term conditions is being discussed.

The National Patient Safety Agency (NPSA) produces guidance on safe medicines practice which can be obtained from its website: www.npsa.nhs.

uk. This Government body also produces alerts which are circulated to all healthcare institutions. These alerts are produced to warn institutions when a series of errors have been made or when potential dangers have been identified. One example is errors made in the administration of oral medicines into vascular access devices. This led to a directive to only use oral syringes to administer syrups/suspensions orally or via nasogastric tubes. These syringes have been designed to be incompatible with intravenous devices.

The Audit Commission has produced two documents concerned with medicines management, and made recommendations for cost savings, including promoting self-medication for most patients in hospital (Audit Commission, 2001, 2002).

Nursing implications
Keeping abreast of new reports from these bodies will help you to improve practice, maintain patient safety and avoid common errors. Audit Commission reports can be obtained from the websites www.dh.gov.uk/ Home/fs/en and www.audit-commission.gov.uk

How do drugs work?
Annie Law

The use of drugs to treat ailments is not new; for thousands of years, extracts from plants and animals have been used to treat many illnesses and some are still used today, e.g. morphine, salicylates, digitalis (Goodinson, 1986a).

As a nurse, you need to have a basic understanding of how drugs reach their target cells and how they work, in order to understand the impact that normal physiological processes and disease have on drug metabolism and excretion. This section will cover the following aspects of pharmacology:

- Drug distribution.
- Mechanism of drug action.
- Metabolism.
- Excretion.
- Adverse reactions.

Drug distribution

Once a drug enters the circulation, a proportion of it binds to plasma proteins, e.g. albumin, some to specific carrier proteins, and some to erythrocytes and other proteins, but it is only the proportion of drug that remains free in the plasma that reaches its target cells. As the free drug in the plasma leaves the circulation, the proportion of the drug that is bound to plasma proteins is released into the plasma.

This works fine if only one drug is taken at a time, but many drugs compete for binding sites on the plasma proteins and literally knock each other off. This increases the amount of free drug in the plasma, resulting in the drug reaching its target cells sooner and therefore exerting a quicker effect, which in some cases can have serious consequences (Goodinson, 1986a; Nursing Times, 1994a; Shepherd, 2002a).

Examples where this happens include:

- Warfarin is displaced by tolbutamide, leading to an increased risk of haemorrhage.
- Tolbutamide is displaced by salicylates, leading to an increased risk of hypoglycaemia.

Drugs are either water or fat soluble. Those that are fat soluble, e.g. diazepam, are more widely distributed in the body and are able to cross the blood–brain barrier.

Clinical relevance

Any change in the body due to the effects of disease can alter drug distribution and therefore the effect of the drug. For example, gentamicin is extremely water soluble; if there is fluid accumulation, such as ascites, the distribution and hence the effect of gentamicin is altered (John and Stevenson, 1995).

Mechanism of drug action

After the drug has travelled in the circulation to its target cells, how does it work? Drugs exert their effects in the body in several ways:

- They may replace missing substances – in vitamin deficiency, diabetes mellitus and hypothyroidism, for example.
- They may interfere with cell function by either stimulating or reducing the normal activity of messengers from one part of the body to another.
- They act against invading organisms or abnormal cells either by inhibiting multiplication of the organism or by killing it directly, e.g. antibiotics, antiviral and antifungal drugs (*Nursing Times*, 1994a).
- Drug action occurs at the cell membrane level, and drugs are categorised as specific or non-specific.

Specific drugs

Specific drugs are drugs that attach to specific receptors on the surface of the cell membrane (Goodinson, 1986a).

It is known that hormones and neurotransmitters exert their physiological effects, and drugs their pharmacological effects, by attaching to specific receptors on the membrane of the cells they are designed to target. This contact triggers events that result in the desired activity. When making contact with receptors, hormones, neurotransmitters and drugs can act as:

- *Agonists*: These cause an observable response when they bind to a specific receptor on the cell membrane.
- *Partial agonists*: These produce a limited response when they bind to a specific receptor, but at the same time prevent the actions of full agonists.
- *Antagonists*: These do not produce a response when they bind to a specific receptor; instead they prevent the action of agonists.

Once a drug has bound to its specific receptor, there is often an increase in the concentration of an intracellular substance before the response occurs; this substance is known as a second messenger (Goodinson, 1986a; Shepherd, 2002a).

Examples of specific drugs include:

- Adrenaline is a beta-receptor agonist: it stimulates cardiac beta-receptors, causing an increase in heart rate.
- Fentanyl and diamorphine are opioid agonists: they mimic the body's own opioid neurotransmitters (endorphins) and produce their analgesic effect by activating the opioid receptors.
- Atenolol is a beta-receptor antagonist: it blocks cardiac beta-receptors, causing a decrease in heart rate.
- Prazocin and doxazocin block the action of alpha-adrenergic receptors in blood vessels, causing vasodilatation and thereby reducing blood pressure.

(John and Stevenson, 1995; Shepherd, 2002a)

Many drugs are not specific to one receptor and will act at more than one site or subset of receptors; this explains the known side-effects of some drugs.

Examples of specific drugs that act at more than one site include:

- Amitriptyline, a tricyclic antidepressant, blocks both the cholinergic and histamine receptors, causing the side-effects of dry mouth, blurred vision, constipation and drowsiness.
- Beta-blockers can attach to both the beta1-receptors in the heart and beta2-receptors in the lungs, the latter causing the side-effect of bronchoconstriction. These drugs should therefore be avoided in asthmatics.

(John and Stevenson, 1995)

Some drugs compete with each other for receptor sites, or they may potentiate each other's stimulating effect on the body.

Example

If naloxone is given to a patient receiving morphine, the effects of morphine are reversed as naloxone knocks the morphine off its receptor.

(*Nursing Times*, 1994a; Shepherd, 2002a).

Non-specific drugs

Non-specific drug action is not mediated by receptors, but is dependent on other factors, such as:

- Enzyme inhibition.
- Enzyme activation.
- Inhibition of cellular transport processes.
- Physico-chemical properties of the drug.
- Inhibition of biochemical processes.

(Goodinson, 1986a)

Examples of non-specific drugs include:

- Enalapril, ramipril and lisinopril are used in heart failure and hypertension: they act by inhibiting angiotensin-converting enzyme.
- Streptokinase and alteplase (fibrinolytic agents) activate plasminogen to form plasmin, which breaks down thrombi.
- Digoxin inhibits the sodium/potassium pump in the heart. Amlodipine, nifedipine and diltiazem (calcium-channel blockers) reduce smooth muscle contraction by blocking the calcium channels, resulting in relaxation of arteriolar smooth muscle. Lansoprazole, a proton pump inhibitor, inhibits the cellular pump that transports hydrogen ions out of the gastric mucosa.
- Furosemide (frusemide) inhibits electrolyte re-absorption in the ascending limb of the loop of Henle in the kidneys.
- Lactulose draws fluid into the bowel by osmosis.
- Penicillins and cephalosporins interfere with bacterial cell wall synthesis.
- Aminogylcosides and tetracyclines inhibit bacterial protein production.
- Quinolones, e.g. ciprofloxacin, inhibit the enzyme that produces bacterial DNA.

(John and Stevenson, 1995; Shepherd, 2002a)

Drug metabolism

This is the breakdown of drugs into a form that is readily excreted. However, not all drugs are metabolised before excretion: some are excreted unchanged in the urine, e.g. digoxin.

Most drug metabolism is carried out in the liver by enzymes; some metabolism also takes place in the gut lining, kidneys and lungs (Goodinson, 1986b; Shepherd, 2002b).

Why is drug metabolism important?

- Most drug interactions occur during metabolism.
- The drug metabolites can exert a pharmacological effect: some drugs are inactive until metabolism has occurred, e.g. cyclophosphamide and prednisolone.
- The body can only metabolise so much of the drug in a set period of time.
- If the metabolism site becomes saturated, the drug action could be prolonged, causing toxicity.
- Drug metabolism breaks down the drug into a water-soluble form ready for excretion (Goodison, 1986b).
- Some drugs can induce or inhibit the production of enzymes that influence the metabolism not only of that drug but also of other drugs. If the inducing or inhibiting agent is removed, toxicity may occur.

Examples of why drug metabolism is important include:

- Carbamazepine and phenobarbitone induce liver enzyme production, which decreases the effect of warfarin, thereby increasing the risk of thrombosis.
- Phenytoin and carbamazepine enhance the metabolism of oral contraceptives, reducing their effectiveness.
- Barbiturates induce enzymes in several pathways, increasing their own metabolism and also that of drugs such as phenytoin and tricyclic antidepressants.
- Cimetidine, omeprazole and amiodarone inhibit liver enzyme production, which increases the effect of warfarin, thereby increasing the risk of bleeding.

  (Goodinson, 1986b; *Nursing Times*, 1994a; John and Stevenson, 1995; Shepherd, 2002a)

Clinical relevance

A patient who is stable on aminophylline decides to give up smoking. With nicotine no longer present, liver enzyme production reduces, drug metabolism slows and plasma levels of aminophylline increase. This may result in toxicity.

Other factors that affect drug metabolism

- Age – especially important in the elderly and the young.
- Alcohol consumption.
- Diseases that affect liver function – half-life of the drug will be prolonged and the effects of the drug can be prolonged or enhanced.

- Smoking – nicotine induces liver enzyme production.
- Genetic factors – genetic abnormalities in enzyme systems that control drug metabolism can affect responsiveness to drugs, e.g. malignant hyperpyrexia in response to the administration of halothane and suxamethonium (Goodinson, 1986b; John and Stevenson, 1995).

Excretion

Drug that is free in the plasma can be excreted via the kidneys (in urine) or the liver (in bile and subsequently in faeces); this is called plasma clearance. Drugs can also be excreted in saliva and sweat and via the lungs (anaesthetic gases) and in breast milk (Goodinson, 1986b; John and Stevenson, 1995).

Clinical relevance
Excretion of some drugs may discolour urine and faeces. This can cause distress in patients if they are not warned to expect this, particularly if the discoloration is red, as people often mistake this for blood.

What is plasma half-life?

This is the time taken for the plasma concentration of a drug to reduce by 50%. Drugs with a shorter half-life will therefore need to be given more often.

Clinical relevance
- Drugs cleared via the kidneys are cleared in proportion to creatinine clearance, and may therefore accumulate in a patient with renal failure. Examples include aminoglycosides and vancomycin.
- Haemodialysis readily removes water-soluble drugs.
- Peritoneal dialysis readily removes lipid-soluble drugs.

(Goodinson, 1986b)

Why do we need to measure the plasma levels of certain drugs?

Some drugs (e.g. gentamicin, theophylline, digoxin) have a very narrow range of plasma concentration within which they are effective and safe. If the plasma concentration is too high, toxicity can occur; if it is too low the treatment will fail. Plasma levels of many drugs are also influenced by other factors, e.g. hypothyroidism, hypokalaemia and hypercalcaemia (Shepherd, 2002a).

Adverse reactions

An adverse reaction is any response that is unintended and of no benefit to the patient. There are two types of adverse reaction (Shepherd, 2002a):

- Type A/augmented reactions: These are related to the normal action of the drug, and are often caused by affinity to more than one type of receptor, e.g. the effects of amitriptyline as described earlier.
- Type B/bizarre reactions: These are reactions unrelated to the drug's normal action or dose, and are unpredictable, e.g. anaphylaxis. Some groups of people are at greater risk of adverse drug reactions.

(Kelly, 2001)

Factors that affect drug action

- Pregnancy: Many drugs cross the placenta and may cause congenital abnormalities or affect the growth and functional development of the fetus, e.g. steroids, narcotics and anaesthetics. Drugs such as aspirin given shortly before or during labour can affect labour or the baby after delivery. Consult the relevant appendix in the *British National Formulary* (BNF) for up-to-date information.
- Breastfeeding: Most drugs will be present in breast milk in small amounts and therefore have potential effects on the baby. However, only a few drugs are contraindicated. These include cyclophosphamide, cyclosporin, bromocriptine and lithium. Consult the relevant appendix in the BNF for up-to-date information.
- Young age: Drug distribution, action, metabolism and excretion in neonates, infants and children may differ from that in adults, because of differences in size, proportions and constituents of the body and physiology, hence adverse effects are more likely.
- Old age: Drug distribution, action, metabolism and excretion in older people are influenced by the normal physiological changes that occur with age and result in deterioration in homeostatic mechanisms and organ function and changes in body composition. Coupled with this, there may be multiple pathology that necessitates the taking of multiple drugs, and reduced functional ability, which may affect the administration of drugs.

Kelly (2001) provides a more detailed rationale of adverse drug reactions in these groups. It is well worth a read to increase your understanding of the specific effects.

What are the principles of safe practice for giving medication?

Annie Law

In 1986 the UKCC produced an advisory paper on the administration of medicines, which stated that first-level nurses and midwives should be considered competent to administer medicines on their own, and be responsible for their actions in so doing. Involvement of a second person would need to occur only if a learner was being taught, the patient's condition made it necessary, or in some exceptional circumstances. Healthcare institutions vary in their policies regarding the checking procedures for drugs, and the number of people who should be involved. Children's services often require two people to check drugs before administration, because of the often complex calculations required. In addition, many institutions require two people to check intravenous (IV) and cytotoxic drugs because of the rapid effect of the drug, and the implications should an error occur.

Table 4.1 provides a step-by-step guide to the stages that should be

Table 4.1. Drug administration flow chart	
Action	**Rationale**
Before administration, read prescription chart carefully. Ensure that you know what the drug is for, the usual dose, side-effects, contraindications and any special instructions or precautions	To check that the prescription is written clearly (in indelible ink) and accurately. It is part of the nurse's role to act as the last line of defence against errors. The doctor may have overlooked potential interactions and may have made a mistake in the dose or route (*Nursing Times*, 1994b, NMC, 2008)
If prescription chart is unclear in any way, return to prescriber for clarification	To reduce the risk of error (Dimond, 2004; Nursing Times, 1994b)
Check that the patient's details are clearly written on the chart. If there are patients with the same or similar name, a warning label should be attached to the chart	To provide sufficient information to check that medicines are given to the correct patient
If more than one chart, ensure that charts are clearly marked 1 of 2, or 2 of 2, as appropriate – merge all onto one chart at earliest opportunity	Ensures that everyone is aware of the existence of more than one chart to reduce the risk of missed doses

Check that the patient's weight is clearly written if any medicine is prescribed where the dose is related to weight	
Check each prescribed medication for: • Name of drug • Route of administration • Dose • Start date • Signature of doctor • Any special instructions (e.g. with food) • Time of last administration • Time due for administration (NMC, 2008)	To ensure that the correct drug is given by the correct route in the right dose at the right time. Some drugs, e.g. antibiotics, are only given for a short course; as the nurse administering the drugs you should request a review of the need for a drug if it has been given for longer
Check for any coexisting therapy, particularly in the 'as required' section	To ensure the same drug or constituent of a drug has not been prescribed in more than one section – risk of overdose (NMC 2008)
Check drug against prescription: • Name of drug • Dose of tablet/capsule/syrup, etc • Calculation (if any) • Expiry date (NMC, 2008)	To ensure that correct dose and drug is given
Check patient's identity against prescription chart and name bracelet. Always ask the patient to state their name, address and date of birth; do not ask 'Are you Mr ....', as a confused, hard-of-hearing, or anxious patient may answer yes to this question when it is not his/her identity	To ensure that correct patient receives the correct drug (*Nursing Times*, 1994b; NMC, 2008)
Obtain patient's consent and administer the drug	Patient's consent is required for all treatments (NMC, 2008)
	Table 4.1 continues

Record that the drug has been administered. Where supervising a student in the administration of medicines, you should clearly countersign the signature of the student (NMC, 2008)	To indicate that the drug has been given and to prevent the dose being given again
Record if the drug has not been given for any reason and inform the prescriber	It may be necessary to alter the route of administration or review the need for the drug (NMC, 2008)
Instruction by telephone to administer a previously unprescribed substance is not acceptable (NMC, 2008)	Risk of unclear instructions or misunderstanding. If absolutely necessary, repeat instructions back to prescriber and ensure that you have a second witness; both of you should record the instructions

followed in the checking and administration of medicines.

The NMC (2008) *Standards for Medicine Management* provides the minimum standard of practice and should be used in conjunction with local policies and procedures.

Nurses should incorporate the five 'rights' of drug administration (*Nursing Times*, 1994b) into their practice:

- Use the right drug.
- Give to the right patient.
- Give the right dose.
- Give by the right route.
- Give at the right time.

Some common problems in the administration of medicines

Conflict with prescriber
What would you do if you felt that the dose of a drug that was prescribed for a patient was unusually high, and when you questioned the doctor who had prescribed it he or she confirmed that this was the intended dose? You are personally accountable for your actions: if you are still concerned, you should check with a more senior doctor and seek advice from a pharmacist. Other sources of information that are available to you include the BNF and any local prescribing guidelines (Dimond, 2004).

Illegible writing
You cannot read clearly the name of the drug that has been prescribed,

but it has been administered by several of your colleagues at previous administration times: If you are in any doubt, do not administer the drug, and check with the prescriber, senior doctor or pharmacist first. If you do not check an illegible prescription and an error occurs, you will be equally liable (Dimond, 2004). After checking with the prescriber, always request that the prescription is rewritten. Many institutions clearly state in their drug policies that prescriptions must be written in capital letters in indelible ink.

PRN (as required) medication

These are drugs prescribed by a doctor, but administered to the patient at the nurse's discretion, based on their assessment of the patient. They typically include analgesics, sleeping tablets, indigestion medicines, etc. Often, insufficient information is provided when these drugs are prescribed, such as the maximum amount that can be given in 24 hours and intervals at which they can be given (Dimond, 2004). You must be aware of the limitations of these drugs. You should check not only the time of the last dose, but also the total that has been given in the last 24 hours, e.g. a patient prescribed paracetamol 1g, which can be given every 4–6 hours, with a maximum of 4g in 24 hours. If the patient requests pain relief at 06.00 hrs, 10.00 hrs, 14.00 hrs and 18.00 hrs, the 24-hour limit will have been reached and if the patient requests further doses, he/she will have received an overdose. When administering drugs prescribed on the PRN part of the prescription chart, you should always check the regularly prescribed drugs to be certain that there are no contraindications. An example of this would be the prescribing of PRN paracetamol and a regular prescription for co-codamol, which could result in an overdose of paracetamol being administered.

Remote orders

The NMC (2008) states that

> *In exceptional circumstances, where medication (NOT including controlled drugs) has been previously prescribed and the prescriber is unable to issue a new prescription, but where changes to the dose are considered necessary, the use of information technology (IT) (such as fax, text message or email) may be used but must confirm any change to the original prescription.*

The NMC makes it clear that if a medication has not been previously prescribed, remote prescribing is not permitted if the prescriber has not assessed the patient, except in life-threatening situations. The key points to remember are:

- A verbal order is not acceptable on its own.
- The fax/email must be stapled to the patient's drug chart.

A new prescription must be signed by the prescriber who sent the fax/ email within 24 hours

A dose is missed

If a dose is missed, for whatever reason, this should be recorded and reported as soon as possible. The implications for a missed dose are:

- Recurrence of symptoms.
- Lower plasma levels of the drug.
- Diminished effect of the drug.

This is especially important for drugs such as insulin, anticoagulants, and drugs for epilepsy, myasthenia gravis and Parkinson's disease (*Nursing Times*, 1994b). Some of the most common reasons for missing a dose are:

- Nil by mouth.
- Nausea/vomiting.
- Patients state that they do not require the drug.

Some drugs can still be administered when the patient is nil by mouth before surgery or a procedure; advice should be sought about which drugs can be given, or they should be administered when the patient returns from the procedure. If the patient is unable to take anything orally for a longer period of time, the need for an alternative route of administration should be discussed with the prescriber.

If patients state that they do not require the drug, an assessment should be made as to whether the drug should be changed to a PRN prescription or whether the patient requires educating about the need to take the drug regularly for maximum benefit. A common example is a patient who stops taking lactulose as soon as they have had their bowels open, and then restart it when they have not had their bowels open for 3–4 days. These patients will require educating about the need to take lactulose regularly and be shown how the daily dose can be titrated until a regular pattern of bowel action is achieved.

Hazardous drugs

Drugs are not without risk to the person administering them and you need to be aware of specific hazards and how you can minimise the risk to yourself. Drugs can present a hazard to the person preparing or administering them through dermal contact, inhalation or inadvertent ingestion (Worthington, 2002).

Hazardous drugs, as defined by Worthington (2002), are drugs that:

- Cause cancer.
- Damage the developing fetus (teratogenic) or impair fertility.
- Cause chromosomal breakage.
- Produce serious organ toxicity at low doses.

The main groups of hazardous drugs (Worthington, 2002) are:

- Cytotoxic drugs.
- Antiviral agents.
- Sex steroid hormones.
- Immunosuppressive drugs.
- Anaesthetic gases.

The above list indicates those drugs which are particularly hazardous; however, repeated exposure to any drug can present a hazard to the nurse. It is therefore vital that you adhere to safe handling practices, not only to protect yourself from harm, but also to prevent you becoming sensitive or resistant to the drugs.

Safe handling practices

- Hazardous drugs should be prepared as much as possible in a properly functioning biological safety cabinet by properly trained staff.
- Always wear protective clothing – gloves when handling any drugs, and aprons, goggles and masks as required.
- Dispose of hazardous drugs in leak-free containers.
- Ensure that you receive proper training in dealing with spillage.
- If using aerosolised hazardous drugs, ensure adequate ventilation and respiratory protection for healthcare workers (Worthington, 2002).
- Never handle tablets because of the risk of sensitisation (*Nursing Times*, 1994b).
- Never eat or drink in drug preparation areas.
- Always wear protective clothing when handling body waste, as some hazardous drugs can be still be present in body fluids several weeks after administration.

What do I need to know about drug calculations?
Annie Law

The calculations that nurses are required to do in relation to drug administration can be complicated, and often cause anxiety. You should be able to make calculations without the use of a calculator, since reliance on a calculator can result in errors. You should always calculate a rough estimate before using a calculator. 'Complex calculations may require a second practitioner to check to minimise the risk of error. Use of calculators should not act as a substitute for arithmetical knowledge and skill' (NMC, 2008).

When two people are involved in the calculations, each should make the calculation separately and agree on the result to minimise the risk of error. The following are a few simple formulae to assist you in the more common calculations, followed by a series of questions for you to test yourself (the answers are provided at the end of the section).

Manually controlled infusions

You do not have a pump to administer an infusion of 1 litre of 0.9% sodium chloride over 6 hours, and need to be able to set the correct rate of drops per minute.

Rate = 'volume' (in drops) divided by 'time' (in minutes)

To be able to calculate the rate, you need to know how many drops per millilitre the administration set delivers. The information can usually be found on the packet, but a rule of thumb would be:

Clear fluids = 20 drops/ml
Blood = 15 drops/ml

To calculate the volume in drops, you need to multiply the volume (in ml) to be administered by the number of drops per ml; to calculate the time in minutes, you need to multiply the time over which the fluid has to be administered by 60, the number of minutes in an hour. The formula therefore becomes:

$$\text{Rate} = \frac{\text{volume (in ml)}}{\text{time (in hours)}} \times \frac{\text{no. of drops per ml}}{60 \text{ (no of minutes in an hour)}}$$

So, if we take the above example of 1 litre of saline over 6 hours:

Rate = $\dfrac{1000 \times 20}{6 \times 60}$ = $\dfrac{20000}{360}$ = $\dfrac{500}{9}$ = 55.55

You would therefore round up the result to 56 drops per minute.

Mechanically controlled infusions

You have a volumetric pump to administer an infusion of 1 litre of 0.9% sodium chloride over 6 hours, and need to be able to set the correct rate of ml per hour.

Rate = volume (in ml) ÷ time (in hours)

So, taking the above example of 1 litre of saline over 6 hours:

Rate = 1000 ÷ 6 = 166.66...

You would therefore round up the result to 167ml per hour.

Sometimes, especially when administering antibiotics, you have to administer smaller amount over periods such as half an hour, 20 minutes or 100 minutes. If we have 100ml to administer over 30 minutes, this is relatively simple, since we know that 30 minutes = 0.5 hour:

Rate = 100 ÷ 0.5 = 200ml per hour

But what if we have 250ml to administer over 100 minutes?

Rate = $\dfrac{\text{volume to be administered (in ml)}}{\text{time (in minutes)}}$ x 60 (minutes in an hour)

= $\dfrac{250 \times 60}{100}$ = 150ml per hour

Drug dose calculations

We often have to administer IV drugs where the dose is different from the amount in the ampoule, and we need to calculate the amount we need to draw up. For example, we need to administer 320mg of gentamicin, which is manufactured in ampoules of 80mg in 2ml. The formula for this type of calculation is:

Amount (in ml) = $\dfrac{\text{what you want}}{\text{what you have got}}$ x what it is in

What you want = 320mg
What you've got = 80mg
What it is in = 2ml
Therefore the calculation is: (320 ÷ 80) x 2 = 8ml

Test yourself on the following calculations

Try them without using a calculator first: the answers can be found at the end of the section

---

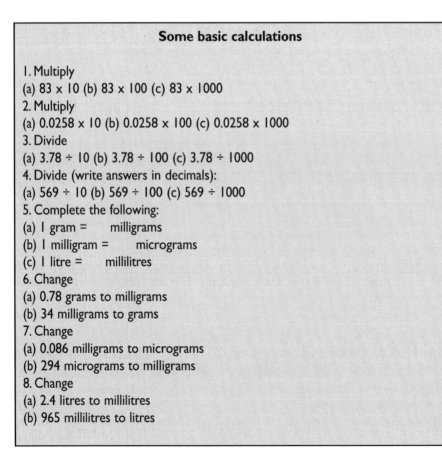

Some basic calculations

1. Multiply
(a) 83 x 10 (b) 83 x 100 (c) 83 x 1000
2. Multiply
(a) 0.0258 x 10 (b) 0.0258 x 100 (c) 0.0258 x 1000
3. Divide
(a) 3.78 ÷ 10 (b) 3.78 ÷ 100 (c) 3.78 ÷ 1000
4. Divide (write answers in decimals):
(a) 569 ÷ 10 (b) 569 ÷ 100 (c) 569 ÷ 1000
5. Complete the following:
(a) 1 gram =   milligrams
(b) 1 milligram =   micrograms
(c) 1 litre =   millilitres
6. Change
(a) 0.78 grams to milligrams
(b) 34 milligrams to grams
7. Change
(a) 0.086 milligrams to micrograms
(b) 294 micrograms to milligrams
8. Change
(a) 2.4 litres to millilitres
(b) 965 millilitres to litres

Drug doses for injection

1. An injection of morphine 8mg is required. Ampoules on hand contain 10mg in 1ml. What volume should be drawn up for injection?
2. Digoxin ampoules on hand contain 500 micrograms in 2ml. What volume is needed to give 350 micrograms?
3. A patient is ordered 16mmol of potassium chloride. Stock solution contains potassium chloride 25mmol in 10ml. What volume is needed?
4. A patient is to be given erythromycin 120mg by injection. Stock vials contain 300mg/10ml. Calculate the required volume.
5. Stock heparin has a strength of 5000units/ml. What volume must be drawn up to give 6500units?
6. Pethidine 85mg is to be given intramuscularly as a premedication. Stock ampoules contain pethidine 100mg in 2ml. Calculate the volume required.
7. A patient is to receive an injection of gentamicin 350mg. IV ampoules on hand contain 80mg/2ml. Calculate the volume required.
8. A patient is prescribed bumetanide 0.8mg intramuscularly. Stock ampoules contain 2mg/4ml. What volume should be drawn up for injection?
9. Folinic acid 365mg is ordered. Stock on hand contains 400mg in 8ml. What volume is required?
10. Stock calciparine contains 25 000 units in 1ml. Calciparine 15 000 units are ordered. What volume is required?

Doses of tablets

1. A patient is ordered co-trimoxazole 960mg orally. Stock on hand is 480mg tablets. Calculate the number of tablets required.
2. How many 30mg tablets of codeine are needed for a dose of 0.06g?
3. A patient is ordered ranitidine 225mg orally. In the ward are 150mg tablets. How many tablets should be given?
4. Ordered: codeine 15mg orally. Stock on hand: codeine tablets 30mg. How many tablets should the patient take?
5. Penicillin 625mg is required. On hand are tablets of strength 250mg. How many tablets should be given?
6. A patient is prescribed 75mg soluble aspirin. On hand are 300mg tablets. How many tablets should be given?
7. Ordered: 0.25mg digoxin orally. Digoxin is available in tablets containing 125 micrograms. How many such tablets should the patient be given?
8. Captopril 25mg is prescribed. How many 50mg tablets should be given?

Doses of syrups/suspensions

In each of the following examples you are given the prescribed dose and the strength of stock mixture on hand. Calculate the volume to be given.

1. Ordered: ampicillin 500mg   On hand: syrup 125mg/5ml
2. Ordered: chloral hydrate 1500mg   On hand: mixture 1g/10ml
3. Ordered: chloramphenicol 750 mg   On hand: suspension 125mg/5ml
4. Ordered: trimethoprim 200mg   On hand: mixture 50mg/5ml
5. Ordered: erythromycin 1250mg   On hand: suspension 250mg/5ml
6. Ordered: aspirin 900mg   On hand: mixture 150mg/5ml
7. Ordered: penicillin 1000mg   On hand: mixture 250mg/5ml
8. Ordered: chlorpromazine 35mg   On hand: syrup 25mg/5ml
9. Ordered: penicillin 1200mg   On hand: mixture 250mg/5ml
10. Ordered: erythromycin 800mg   On hand: mixture 125mg/5ml

Infusion rates

1. A patient is to have 800ml Hartmann's solution over 10 hours. The IV set delivers 15 drops/ml. Calculate the rate in drops/min.
2. 325ml of blood is to be given over 4 hours. The IV set delivers 15 drops/ml. Calculate the rate in drops/min.
3. 800ml of fluid is to drip at 50 drops/min. How long will the fluid last if the IV set delivers 15 drops/ml?
4. Half a litre of fluid is being given at 25 drops/min. The IV set delivers 15 drops/ml. What time will it take to give this amount?

Answers

Basic calculations
(1a) 830 (1b) 8300 (1c) 83000; (2a) 0.258 (2b) 2.58 (2c) 25.8.
(3a) 0.378 (3b) 0.0378 (3c) 0.00378; (4a) 56.9 (4b) 5.69 (4c) 0.569
(5a) 1000 (5b) 1000 (5c) 1000; (6a) 780mg (6b) 0.034g; (7a) 86 μg (7b) 0.294mg
(8a) 2400ml (8b) 0.965 litres
Drug doses for injection
(1) 0.8 ml; (2) 1.4 ml; (3) 6.4 ml; (4) 4 ml; (5) 1.3 ml; (6) 1.7 ml; (7) 8.75 ml; (8) 1.6 ml; (9) 7.3 ml; (10) 0.6 ml
Doses of tablets
(1) 2; (2) 2; (3) 1.5; (4) 0.5; (5) 2.5; (6) 0.25; (7) 2; (8) 0.5
Doses of syrups/suspensions
(1) 20ml; (2) 15ml; (3) 30ml; (4) 20ml; (5) 25ml; (6) 30ml; (7) 20ml; (8) 7ml; (9) 24ml; (10) 32ml
Infusion rates
(1) 20 drops/min; (2) 20 drops/min; (3) 4 hours; (4) 5 hours

What are the routes of drug administration?
Annie Law

The manner in which drugs are administered determines whether the patient benefits from the treatment or suffers adverse effects. Examples include:

- Furosemide (frusemide) given too quickly intravenously can cause deafness.
- Oral penicillin given with food is not well absorbed.
- Over-application of topical steroids causes thinning of the skin, which increases absorption and leads to systemic side-effects (Shepherd, 2002b).

Two factors determine whether the drug will reach its intended site of action in the body:

- Bioavailability of the drug.
- How the drug is administered.

Bioavailability

This is the proportion of the drug that enters the systemic circulation and reaches the site of action. If administered by the IV route, 100% bioavailability is achieved. Although some drugs administered orally (e.g. ciprofloxacin) are well absorbed and achieve a bioavailability similar to that achieved by the IV route, most drugs given orally do not and require an oral dose significantly higher than their IV dose. One of the reasons for this is that first-pass metabolism occurs with oral drug administration. Drugs are absorbed across the intestinal mucosa and enter the portal circulation; they then pass through the liver, where a proportion of the drug is metabolised, reducing its bioavailability. Some enzymatic breakdown also occurs in the intestinal mucosa and lungs (Goodinson, 1986a; *Nursing Times*, 1994b; John and Stevenson, 1995; Shepherd, 2002b). Some drugs, e.g. gentamicin, do not easily cross the gastrointestinal tract mucosa and oral absorption does not occur (John and Stevenson, 1995). An example is:

- The beta-blocker propranolol is given in a dose of 40mg or above orally, but in a dose of only 1mg intravenously.

Oral drug administration

This is the most frequently used route, the most convenient and the most economical. The solid forms of oral preparation are very stable and the dose is accurate. Absorption from the gastrointestinal tract occurs mostly in the small intestine where the surface area is greatest.

The oral route, however, is not without problems and many factors can make absorption from the gastrointestinal tract unpredictable. For example, the presence of food in the gastrointestinal tract can alter:

- pH.
- Gut motility – increased motility means less time available for absorption.
- Emptying time of the stomach – if emptying time is delayed, the drug will not reach the intestine and the rate of absorption will therefore be reduced.
- Rate and extent of drug absorption:
  - cephalexin, amoxycillin and isoniazid are less well absorbed in the presence of food
  - flucloxacillin taken on a full stomach will only achieve 30–50% absorption and should therefore be given 1 hour before food or on an empty stomach
  - tetracycline is less well absorbed in the presence of dairy products
  - other drugs, such as aspirin and prednisolone, should be given with or after food to decrease gastric irritation.

(Goodinson, 1986a; John and Stevenson, 1995; *Nursing Times*, 1994b; Shepherd, 2002a, 2002b)

Malabsorption syndromes such as Crohn's or coeliac disease can either increase or decrease drug absorption. Absorption may be reduced if a patient has diarrhoea or constipation.

The patient may be unable to swallow tablets or capsules. In this situation, there are a few options available:

- Some tablets can be broken into smaller pieces or crushed. Some are specifically designed to dissolve or to be chewed. Enteric-coated or sustained-release tablets should never be crushed or chewed as this damages the release-controlling mechanism, resulting in the whole dose being absorbed at once rather than over a number of hours. Toxicity or overdose may occur if the whole dose is absorbed at once, and suboptimal treatment will result if the dose is not absorbed at all (*Nursing Times*, 1994b; John and Stevenson, 1995; Shepherd, 2002b).
- Some capsules can be opened and the contents sprinkled onto food or mixed with a small amount of water.
- Many drugs are available as syrups or in dispersible form.
- Caution should be taken to ensure that patients do not leave tablets to

dissolve in the mouth if they are intended to be swallowed whole, as this could cause burns to the oral mucosa.

Nursing implications

Timing of drug administration is important to ensure optimum treatment, especially when the drug must be given before or with food.

- Always seek advice from a pharmacist regarding the crushing, chewing or opening of capsules.
- Tablets containing drugs that are gastric irritants are enteric coated so that the tablet remains intact in the stomach before passing into the small intestine, where the coating is dissolved. Patients should not take antacids that alter the gastric pH at the same time as enteric-coated tablets as the coating may dissolve in the stomach, causing irritation and ulceration of the gastric mucosa (John and Stevenson, 1995; Strachan, 2001; Shepherd, 2002a), diarrhoea or constipation (John and Stevenson, 1995).

Sublingual drug administration

This is not a common route; perhaps the most well-known drug to be administered this way is glyceryl trinitrate (GTN) for angina. The tablet is placed under the tongue and allowed to dissolve. The drug is rapidly absorbed into the systemic circulation and avoids first-pass metabolism in the liver (*Nursing Times*, 1994b; John and Stevenson, 1995; Shepherd, 2002b).

Rectal drug administration

This route also avoids first-pass metabolism in the liver. The benefits include:

- Valuable means of localised drug delivery to the large bowel, e.g. rectal steroids for the treatment of ulcerative colitis or Crohn's disease.
- Delivery of antiemetics in a patient who is unable to take oral drugs because of nausea and/or vomiting.
- Delivery of drugs in a patient who is unable to swallow.
- Delivery of drugs that could be inactivated by gastric secretions.
                    (Goodinson, 1986a; *Nursing Times*, 1994b; Shepherd, 2002b)

Nursing implications
- Some people find the rectal route unacceptable – you should check its acceptability with the patient.

- The presence of hard faeces in the rectum will affect the absorption of a drug by this route; drugs should be placed against the mucosa and not in the centre of faeces.
- Rectal administration should be avoided in patients:
  - with a low platelet count – risk of bleeding
  - with neutropenia – risk of mobilising bacteria
  - who have recently undergone rectal and/or anal surgery.
- Caution should be taken in patients with large haemorrhoids.
- Correct storage of rectal drugs is important as suppositories may melt at high temperatures.

    (John and Stevenson, 1995; *Nursing Times*, 1994b; Shepherd, 2002b)

Topical drug administration

This is the direct application of drugs to the tissues to treat localised disease. Advantages include:

- Drug availability at the intended site of action.
- Reduced systemic side-effects.

    Examples of topical drug administration include:

- Ointments/creams to the skin.
- Eye drops.
- Nose drops.
- Ear drops.
- Inhaled bronchodilators.
- Vaginal pessaries.

Topical administration can also be used to deliver drugs to the systemic circulation, usually over a sustained period of time – in some cases several weeks. This is achieved via transdermal patches. Drugs administered by this route include GTN, fentanyl and hormones (*Nursing Times*, 1994b; John and Stevenson, 1995; Shepherd, 2002b).

Nursing implication
- Always wear gloves when applying topical preparations to reduce the risk of absorption through your skin (John and Stevenson, 1995).

Parenteral drug administration

This includes subcutaneous (SC), intramuscular (IM) and intravenous (IV) drug administration. All of these routes avoid first-pass metabolism in the liver (Goodinson, 1986a).

Subcutaneous and intramuscular drug administration

These routes allow a 'depot' of a drug to be inserted into the muscle or adipose tissue, from where the drug is released into the systemic circulation over time and achieves a slow, sustained action. Some oil-based injections given this way need only be administered monthly or even 3-monthly (Shepherd, 2002b).

Nursing implications
- The patient must be assessed for suitability for these routes, as the state of the patient, e.g. presence of shock or oedema, can sometimes lead to unpredictable absorption.
- The nurse must be aware of the underlying structures, such as nerves, which can be accidentally hit if the drug is not injected in the correct place.
- Knowledge of the correct technique and placement is paramount.
- Avoid SC or IM injections in patients with:
  - liver disease
  - clotting abnormalities
  - low platelet counts.

(John and Stevenson, 1995)

Sites for SC injection
- Outer aspect of the upper arm.
- Mid-abdominal wall.
- Outer aspect of the thigh.

(Gilsenan, 2000)

SC injections are traditionally given at a 45° angle, but with the new shorter needles, such as those used for insulin injection, a 90° angle should be used. The skin should be pinched to lift the adipose tissue away from the muscle, as inadvertent injection into the muscle will result in more rapid absorption of the drug. It is not necessary to aspirate the needle after insertion into SC tissue; in fact, aspiration before the administration of heparin increases the risk of haematoma (Workman, 1999).

Sites for IM injection
- Deltoid muscle of the upper arm.
- Gluteus maximus muscle.
- Gluteus medius muscle.
- Anterior quadriceps muscle.

(Workman, 1999; Gilsenan, 2000)

It is important to inject the drug into a well-perfused muscle to ensure rapid systemic action. Patient assessment will influence the choice of site and should include:

- Patient's general status – muscle mass.
- Patient's age.
- Amount of drug to be given.

Sites should be rotated if repeated injections are required. The needle should be inserted at a 90° angle and aspirated for 5–10 seconds to check that a blood vessel has not been accessed; discard if blood is obtained. Inject slowly approximately 1ml every 10 seconds to allow the muscle fibres to expand and absorb the drug. Wait 10 seconds before withdrawing the needle, to allow the drug to diffuse into the muscle. Do not massage the site as this encourages the drug to leak out (Beyea and Nicoll, 1996; Workman, 1999).

Complications of IM injections include:

- Pain.
- Muscle atrophy.
- Fibrosis.
- Nerve damage.
- Tissue necrosis.
- Gangrene.

(Workman, 1999)

Nursing implication

Regular swabbing of the skin with alcohol before subcutaneous or intramuscular injections can result in hardening of the skin. If the patient is physically clean and the nurse has maintained a high standard of hand hygiene and asepsis throughout, there is no need to clean the skin. However, if you do clean the skin, you should allow 30 seconds for it to dry as injection of alcohol causes a stinging sensation (Workman, 1999).

Intravenous (IV) drug administration

This route should only be used if no alternative route is available, since it is the most inconvenient route for both the patient and the practitioner. It also carries the greatest risk of all the routes of administration, owing to:

- The immediate onset of action.
- The often complex calculations.
- The often complex dilutions.

- The need for extra care with administration rates, e.g. furosemide (frusemide) should not exceed 4mg/min to prevent transient hearing loss; vancomycin should not exceed 10mg/min to reduce the risk of hypotension, shock and cardiac arrest.
- Possible incompatibilities with other IV solutions.
- Use of infusion devices.
- Risk of infection – aseptic technique required.
- Harm to patient from extravasation.

(John and Stevenson, 1995; Shepherd 2002b)

Protein preparations should not be shaken, but should be rotated gently to prevent denaturation and frothing (*Nursing Times*, 1994b).

Nursing implications

- Most NHS trusts require practitioners to undergo additional training before allowing them to administer IV drugs.
- You should ensure that before administering any IV drug, you are knowledgeable about the action of the drug, its side-effects, and whether dilution is required before administration. Some drugs can cause severe phlebitis if not diluted adequately before administration.
- You should also be aware of the guidance provided by the NMC (2008) and ensure that, if you are administering the drug, you have either prepared it yourself or witnessed the preparation: 'Registrants must not prepare substances for injection in advance of their immediate use or administer medication drawn into a syringe or container by another practitioner when not in their presence.'
- Exceptions to this include an already established infusion, and medications prepared in pharmacy and labelled for an individual patient.

What are the ethical issues in drug administration?
Annie Law

When patients refuse their drugs, nurses face a dilemma: should they disguise the medicines in food or drink or just not give the medication, which might result in deterioration of the patient's health? Is covert administration ethical or legal? This method of administration has been common practice over the years in many settings where the nurse is acting alone. The NMC (2007) produced a statement on disguising medicine in food and drink in an attempt to assist practitioners in decision making. As a registered nurse it is your professional duty to familiarise yourself with this document.

There are ethical, legal and pharmaceutical issues that need to be considered in the covert administration of drugs. Ethically, is it right to trick a patient into taking medication? There may be circumstances when, by so doing, you save a life or avoid substantial harm. If you did administer a medication covertly, can you be prosecuted under criminal law or the Human Rights Act (Treloar et al, 2000, 2001)? The NMC (2007) advises that disguising medicines in the absence of informed consent may be regarded as deception. A clear distinction should always be made between those who have the capacity to refuse medication and whose refusal should be respected, even if the decision adversely affects their health, and those who lack this capacity. The pharmaceutical properties of a drug may be changed if the preparation is crushed and added to food or drink.

Nursing implications
You should never feel that you have to make a decision alone to administer drugs covertly, and it is recommended that you follow the steps outlined below if the patient does not have the capacity to make an informed decision:

- Discuss with the multiprofessional team.
- Discuss with the patient's relatives.
- Respect any previous instruction left by the patient.
- Consult local policies or, if not available, ask to see them.
- Seek advice from your employer's legal advisors.
- Maintain good records of decisions and actions taken.
- Agree a method of administration with the pharmacist.
- Remember that the capacity to consent can fluctuate and should be regularly reassessed.
- Remember that you are accountable for your actions.

(NMC, 2007)

How can I avoid drug errors?
Annie Law

> *It is worth bearing in mind that administering drugs in a busy ward can be rather like driving, in that it is easy to allow a sense of routine to take over and not concentrate fully on the job in hand. Like driving, mistakes can happen at any time, and they may prove fatal.*
>
> (*Nursing Times*, 1994b)

Lack of knowledge is a common cause of error (Cavell, 2000); however, care also needs to be taken when two patients have the same or a similar name.

There are two main types of error (*Nursing Times*, 1994b):

- Error of omission: Where the nurse unintentionally fails to give a prescribed drug.
- Error of commission: Where the nurse administers a drug that was not prescribed, or an excessive dose of a prescribed drug.

In the past, drug errors were often linked with blame and led to disciplinary action. This led to fear of reporting errors and the potential harm to patients going unchecked (Department of Health, 2000a). Today the NHS promotes an 'open, no blame' culture to encourage reporting. All incidents, however, do require a thorough investigation to be able to distinguish between errors that were concealed or occurred as a result of reckless or incompetent practice, and those that occurred as a result of pressure of work and where there was immediate, honest disclosure in the patient's interest (NMC, 2008). The Government document *An Organisation with a Memory* (Department of Health, 2000a) identified common errors that have resulted in litigation claims. They include:

- Incorrect or inappropriate drugs.
- Wrong drug.
- Administration error.
- Failure to warn the patient of the side-effects.

The National Patient Safety Agency (NPSA) has been charged with the task of ensuring that reporting of errors, and lessons learnt from them, are disseminated throughout the NHS (Shepherd, 2002c).

Risk management strategies use 'near misses' as a way of reducing systemic errors, such as ensuring that sufficient information is available to prescribers, promoting electronic prescribing to reduce the risk of errors from poor handwriting, and integrating pharmacists into clinical teams to anticipate errors rather than discover them (Cavell and Hughes, 1997; Audit Commission, 2001).

Nursing implications

You can avoid making drug errors by following some simple principles:

- Always check the prescription carefully against the drug to be administered.
- Always check the patient's identity against the prescription chart, even if it is your own mother or a patient you have known for many years.
- Be assertive to prevent interruptions during the drug administration process; wait until you have finished.
- Always follow local policies and procedures; they are there to protect the patient from harm and yourself from errors.
- If you do make an error, report it immediately to minimise harm to the patient.

What are the alternative and new initiatives in drug administration?

Annie Law

Self-administration

Receiving medication from the nurse by the traditional drug round method while in hospital encourages dependent behaviour in patients, and rarely includes education of patients about their drugs (Leadbeater, 1991). If patients are not fully informed about their medications they are unlikely to comply fully. This could result in:

- Slower recovery from illness.
- Increased risk of secondary health problems.
- Poorer quality of life.
- Deterioration in the patient's condition.
- Re-admission to hospital.
- Premature death.

(Williams, 1991; Shepherd, 2002c)

The reasons why patients fail to comply include:

- Forgetting to take the occasional tablet.
- Taking too high a dose.
- Failing to get the prescription dispensed, because of apathy, lack of understanding of why the medications have been prescribed, or inability to pay for the prescription.
- Feeling better and ceasing to take the drug before the end of a course.
- Undesirable side-effects.
- Complexity of the regimen – multiple drugs.
- A behaviour change is required while taking the drugs, such as no alcohol or dietary restrictions.

(Williams, 1991; Shepherd, 2002c)

Compliance can be improved by:

- Counselling and education.
- Assessment of the patient's ability to administer the drugs.
- Provision of aids to facilitate administration, e.g. easy-to-open bottles, measuring cups and spoons, dosette boxes.
- Providing adequate information about each drug.

(Williams, 1991; Shepherd, 2002c)

Self-administration by patients or carers while in hospital is supported by the NMC (2004) and the Audit Commission (2001), and fits in with the philosophy of self-care and patient education. The advantages of self-administration are:

- Enables patients to become responsible for their drugs in preparation for discharge, while having access to professional support.
- Improves patients' knowledge of their drugs.
- Increases compliance.
- Improves communication between the patient and the nurse.
- Enables patients to keep to their home routine and usual times, e.g. being able to take their medication with food, or at night, without having to wait for the drug round.

(Leadbeater 1991, Shepherd 2002b, 2002c)

Self-medication is not just a matter of handing the drugs over to the patient or carer; it requires a change in your role in the drug administration process – from one of administering to one of assessing, supervising and educating.

Nursing implications
- If patients are not going to administer their own medicines on discharge from hospital, they will not be suitable for self-administration in hospital.
- Patients should be assessed for their suitability to administer their medicines, including manual dexterity and memory – aids could be utilised if any difficulties are identified. Discuss with your pharmacist.
- Patients' competence should be reviewed periodically.
- Use patients' own medicines wherever possible, as patients will already be familiar with the packaging and names.
- Medication for self-administration should be labelled with the patient's name and clear instructions on how and when to take the drugs.
- Complete any documentation that your institution requires – this may be in the form of a consent form or disclaimer. A record should be made in patients' care plans that they are self-administering.
- Patients should be supplied with a record card that contains all details of the medicine to be taken, including:
  - name of the drug
  - purpose
  - how the drug should be taken
  - when it should be taken
  - how long it should be taken for
  - any special precautions or storage requirements
  - side-effects.

- You should check, on a daily basis or more often if required, that patients are administering their medicines correctly, and keep a record of this checking procedure.
- The patient's drug chart should be clearly marked that the patient is self-administering to ensure that any change to regimen is communicated promptly to the nurse and the patient.
- If any changes are made to the prescription, the patient will require educating about the additions. If any drugs are discontinued, these should be removed from the patient's bedside immediately.
- You should ensure that patients are aware of their responsibility for the safety and secure storage of their medicines, which should be kept in a locked cupboard or drawer at their bedside.

(Leadbeater, 1991; Shepherd 2002b, 2002c)

Patient group directions

Many clinic areas used to have 'standing orders' – a list of drugs that a nurse could administer to a patient without a doctor's prescription. However, the Crown Report (Department of Health, 1999) showed that these had no legal standing. This led to the publication of a new statutory instrument (Department of Health, 2000b), which introduced patient group directions (PGDs).

What are PGDs?

PGDs are 'written instructions for the supply or administration of medicines to groups of patients who may not be individually identified before presentation for treatment' (Department of Health, 2000b).

This is not nurse prescribing and should not be confused with it.

Why do we need PGDs?

PGDs are needed to improve services to patients: they reduce delays in treatment by ensuring that the right treatment is delivered by the right professional at the right time. Patient choice should be taken into account: if patients prefer to wait for a prescription from a doctor, that choice should be respected (Spyropoulos, 2002).

How do I know what I can administer?

The legislation is very clear about how a PGD should be produced and what it should include:

- The name of the business to which the direction applies, e.g the ward within a hospital.
- The date the direction comes into force and the date it expires.
- Class of health professional who may supply or administer the medicine.

- Signature of the doctor/dentist and pharmacist who have agreed to the direction.
- Signature of the appropriate representative of the organisation.
- Description of the medicine to which the direction applies.
- Clinical condition or situation to which the direction applies.
- Description of those patients excluded from being treated under the direction.
- Description of the circumstances in which further advice should be sought from a doctor and arrangements made for referral.
- Details of appropriate dosage and maximum total dose, quantity, pharmaceutical form and strength, route and frequency of administration.
- Relevant warnings, including potential adverse reactions.
- Details of any necessary follow-up actions and the circumstances.
- A statement of the records to be kept for audit purposes.

(Department of Health, 2000b)

Are there any drugs that cannot be included under a PGD?
Yes - controlled drugs cannot be used with a PGD.

Can any nurse supply or administer the medicines included within a PGD?
No – only fully competent, trained professionals can operate within a PGD (Spyropoulos, 2002). Most organisations require a nurse to undertake additional training before she/he can operate within a PGD. You should check the requirements of your own trust.

Nurse prescribing

This section provides only a brief summary of nurse prescribing since the nurse is expected to have several years of experience in the clinical specialty and be practising at a senior level before being able to undertake this role. In 1992 the Medicinal Products: Prescribing by Nurses Etc. Act was passed. This was amended in 1994 to provide a revised list of products in the Nurse Prescriber's formulary, which applied only to community nurses.

In 1999 the Crown report recommended that prescribing authority was extended to other first level nurses.

In 2001 the Department of Health produced an extended formulary that included:

- All general sales list
- All pharmacy medicines

- Some prescription only medicines to enable nurses to prescribe in four areas:
  - minor ailments
  - minor injuries
  - health promotion
  - palliative care.

In 2002 education and training commenced providing a comprehensive programme over a 3-month period. This included 25 taught days accompanied by learning in practice supported and assessed by a mentor. Since nurse prescribers are accountable both legally and professionally they have to possess greater knowledge of pharmacokinetics, pharmacodynamics, anatomy, physiology, the disease process and the patient's circumstances, past medical history and current medications (Courtenay and Butler, 2002).

In 2003 the regulations were amended to include Supplementary Prescribing. This allows nurses who undergo a similar course as the Independent Prescribing curriculum, to prescribe from the medical formulary (with the exception of controlled drugs). Before this can happen a management plan needs to be written in conjunction with the supplementary prescriber, the medical practitioner and the patient. In 2006 Nurse Independent Prescribing discontinued the extended formulary and qualified nurse independent prescribers (formerly known as extended formulary nurse prescribers) are now able to prescribe any licensed medicine for any medical condition within their competence, including some controlled drugs. Currently there is consultation ongoing on whether some nurse prescribers, particularly palliative care nurses, can prescribe medicines to be administered in an unlicensed form if this is deemed standard practice. An example would be the mixing of medicines in a syringe driver for subcutaneous administration. This new initiative will be of particular benefit for patients with chronic medical conditions.

Your status as a nurse prescriber must be recorded on the NMC register (NMC, 2004).

References

Audit Commission (2001) *A Spoonful of Sugar: Medicines management in NHS hospitals*. Audit Commission, London

Audit Commission (2002) *Review of National Findings: Medicines management*. Audit Commission, London

Beyea SC, Nicoll LH (1996) Administering IM injections the right way. *Americal Journal of Nursing* **96**(1): 34–5

Cavell G (2000) Drugs: The nurse's responsibility. *Professional Nurse* **15**(5): 296

Cavell G, Hughes DK (1997) Does computerised prescribing improve the accuracy of drug administration? *Pharmaceutical Journal* **259**: 782–4

Courtenay M, Butler M (2002) Education and nurse prescribing. *Nursing Times* **98**(9): 53–54

Department of Health (1999) *Making a Difference: Strengthening the nursing, midwifery and health visiting contribution to health and healthcare* (The Crown Report). HMSO, London

Department of Health (2000a) *An Organisation with a Memory: Report of an expert group on learning from adverse events in the NHS*. The Stationery Office, London

Department of Health (2000b) *Patient Group Directions (England only)*. HSC2000/026. Health & Safety Commission, London

Department of Health (2001) Patients to get quicker access to medicines. Press release 4.5.2001.Ref 2001/0223. HMSO, London

Department of Health (2009) Guidance Issued to GPs and Oncology Departments Regarding Cancer. Available from: http://www.nhsbsa.nhs.uk/Documents/HealthCosts/Guidance_issued_to_GPs_and_oncology_departments_regarding_cancer [accessed 13.11.2009]

Department of Health/National Practitioner Programme (2006) *A Guide to the Mechanisms for the Prescribing, Supply and Administration of Medicine*. HMSO, London

Dimond B (2004) *Legal Aspects of Nursing*. 4th edn. Prentice Hall, New York

Gilsenan I (2000) A practical guide to giving injections. *Nursing Times* **96**(33): 43–4

Goodinson SM (1986a) Fundamentals of drug action administration and absorption: An overview. *Nursing (Lond)* 3(10): 386–90

Goodinson SM (1986b) Fundamentals of drug action: Drug elimination. *Nursing (Lond)* **3**(12): 466–7

John A, Stevenson T (1995) A basic guide to the principles of drug therapy. *British Journal of Nursing* **4**(20): 1194–8

Kelly J (2001) Minimising potential side-effects of medication at different ages. *Professional Nurse* **17**(4): 259–62

Leadbeater M (1991) Increasing knowledge. *Nursing Times* **87**(30): 32–5

Nursing and Midwifery Council (2004) *Guidelines for the Administration of Medicines*. Nursing and Midwifery Council, London

Nursing and Midwifery Council (2007) *Covert administration of medicines - disguising medicine in food and drink. Advice Sheet* . From: http://www.nmc-uk.org [accessed 18.11.2009]

Nursing and Midwifery Council (2008) *Standards for Medicines Management.* Nursing and Midwifery Council, London

Nursing Times (1994a) Professional development. Medication: knowledge for practice. *Nursing Times* **90**(36 Suppl): 1–4

Nursing Times (1994b) Professional development. Medication: the role of the nurse. *Nursing Times* **90**(37 Suppl): 5–8

Shepherd M (2002a) Medicines 1. Pharmacology. *Nursing Times* **98**(15): 43–6

Shepherd M (2002b) Managing medicines. *Nursing Times* **98**(17): 43–6

Shepherd M (2002c) Managing medicines. *Nursing Times* **98**(17): 43–6

Spyropoulos A (2002) Patient group directions. *Nursing Times* **98**(9): 48

Strachan I (2001) Medicines and older people: A nurse's guide to administration. *British Journal of Community Nursing* **6**(6): 296–301

Treloar A, Beats B, Philpot M (2000) A pill in the sandwich: Covert medication in food and drink. *Journal of the Royal Society of Medicine* **93**(8): 408–11

Treloar A, Philpot M, Beats B (2001) Concealing medicines in patient's food. *Lancet* **357**(9249): 62–4

Williams B (1991) Medication education. *Nursing Times* **87**(29): 50–52

Worthington KA (2002) Hazardous drugs. *American Journal of Nursing* **102**(5): 120

Workman B (1999) Safe injection techniques. *Nursing Standard* **13**(39): 47–53

Notes

CHAPTER 5

The role of the staff nurse

- How do I adjust to becoming a staff nurse?
- How do I work with others and become part of the team?
- How do I manage my time?
- How do I get to grips with working unsocial hours?
- What should I expect from clinical supervision?
- How do I deal with experienced healthcare assistants?
- What am I meant to do on a ward round?
- What do I need to know about the research process?
- How can we begin to evaluate practice?
- What issues are involved in obtaining consent?
- What is involved in professional development?
- How can I develop my professional practice?
- What sort of post-registration course should I do?
- What are CAT points and APAs?
- What is involved in reflective practice?
- How do I prepare for an interview?
- What is the role of the mentor?
- What is involved in teaching a student?
- What is involved in assessing a student?
- What are my roles and responsibilities regarding the Mental Health Act?
- How do I refer patients to the community services?
- How do I refer patients to the multidisciplinary team?
- What are my rights and responsibilities regarding risk management?
- What do I need to know about clinical governance?

How do I adjust to becoming a staff nurse?
Penny Tremayne

Transition: A reality shock

Cast you mind back a few years, can you remember why you wanted to become a nurse? Responses to this question may have included:

- I wanted to make a difference.
- I am a kind and caring person.
- I am a people person.

Hopefully nothing has changed. As a student nurse there is a tendency to wish the time away. However, there is a mixture of emotions when putting on that new uniform; not only are you visible as a registered nurse you are actually one. Even the most confident of student nurses may wish they could reverse time to the safety of being a student once again. Fear, excitement and anxiety are all normal. At university you may recall people harping on about 'lifelong learning' and while you will pursue further education, the learning of 'real-life nursing' begins once you register. A useful analogy is when you learn to drive. You achieve the proficiencies required but it is only through experience that you truly develop and refine those skills and adapt appropriately.

So there are differences; yes, you are now professionally accountable, you do have a uniform and probably greater responsibility in the healthcare setting you are working in but the fundamentals of nursing care have not changed.

What does a ward/unit manager expect of a newly registered nurse? These expectations may be:

- To deliver a high standard of care.
- To be kind and caring to patients, staff and relatives.
- To be honest and trustworthy.
- To communicate effectively.
- To demonstrate initiative and use common sense.
- To priortise workload.
- To be a good team worker.
- To supervise staff, work as a team leader and delegate work appropriately.
- To be punctual, neat and tidy.

Much of this will have been undertaken as a student nurse. You need to be kind to yourself and understand it is normal to be nervous. Locasto and Kochanek (1989) explain a 'reality shock' that nurse educators go through that can be useful to explore to make better sense of what you as a newly registered nurse may also be going through.

In the honeymoon period, as a newly registered nurse, there is a sense of 'novelty'. An end to a bursary/means tested grant results in a salary and some decent money at long last. The hard work of the previous three years has resulted in the ultimate goal and there is a sense of achievement. The work setting welcomes you and you no longer have placements; finally you are part of a team.

Shock and rejection can follow. The shock phase comprises four phases:

- Moral outrage – newly registered nurses can find the intensity of shifts too much, being called to come in on 'days off' to cover for sickness of colleagues. Due to shortage of staff, shifts can become prolonged, and they (the managers) want the nurse to take on different roles – what time will there be to do that?

- Rejection – with all intentions to be the 'best staff nurse' confrontations and frustrations with other staff members and limited resources can make newly registered nurses feel as though they are a failure. There may be a perception that others are much better.
- Fatigue – adapting to the new role can leave newly registered nurses physically and mentally exhausted. Fatigue may impact on their social life leaving them too tired to pursue hobbies and with compromised relationships.
- Perceptual distortion – newly registered nurses can think that they are not working as effectively as other registered nurses and anger can develop towards the healthcare setting that they are working within. This can sometimes be vented at meetings where contributions can be hyper-critical, superficial and lack objectivity. All in all the perception can be all too negative. It is as if newly registered nurses are in 'too deep' and are in a state of 'shock'.
- Resolution – this is the final stage and refers to a sense of recovery or resolution.

Finding a role model, someone who can offer assistance in this difficult time, may be helpful. Although some areas may have a preceptorship programme in place newly registered nurses may seek solace in a person away from the particular setting who may be better able to help them make sense of the situation. One strategy to try and enable newly registered nurses to adapt better may be a reflective diary. In a diary they may be able to identify, develop and change their practices. By adopting such strategies newly registered nurses can begin to lessen the intensity and even see an amusing side to it all, a sense of objectivity will be beginning to dawn.

Benner (1984) identified five levels of competency in clinical nursing practice, namely; novice, advanced beginner, competent, proficient and expert. In this seminal piece of writing Benner (1984) acknowledges the complexity of nursing, and considers that proficient nurses have often worked with a similar patient population for 3–5 years and the expert nurse often has an intuitive grasp of situations. Therefore it is unfair to compare yourself to nurses who are more experienced than yourself.

Realise that becoming newly registered is a transition that can have aspects of the reality shock discussed. Try and put into place strategies that will support you through this time so that the transition you make is less shock and rejection and more honeymoon and resolution. Good luck.

How do I work with others and become part of the team?

Karen Jackson

Becoming part of a team

As a newly qualified nurse, becoming part of a team can be very daunting: everyone else seems to know each other and you are keen to make a good impression. The first time you have to answer the phone and say 'staff nurse' can be frightening as the person on the other end will not necessarily know whether you have been in post 5 minutes or 5 months. These feelings are normal, so what can help you to function effectively?

Remember that people expect you to be asking questions and to be in need of support. A small notebook arranged alphabetically can act as a memory booster and save you having to ask the same questions repeatedly. Find out if your trust or employer offers some kind of preceptorship programme. If so, utilise opportunities to meet with your preceptor to discuss your progress and give you feedback on how you are getting on. If not, is there someone in the area who could act as a buddy and provide you with some support?

You need to spend some time understanding how the team works. This can include finding out about:

- Systems such as team, named or primary nursing.
- Teams of medical staff, which house officers and registrars work for which consultant, and how the on-call system works. This may save you a lot of frustrating phone calls when you need someone to review a patient.
- How to seek help and advice if you are in a patient's home or other non-hospital setting.
- Therapists and other professionals, e.g. pharmacists, attached to the ward or area. You need to know how to contact them: do you need to phone or will they be visiting the ward/area regularly to pick up referrals? What documentation needs to be completed, e.g. referral cards or pharmacy request slips? Are these paper based or electronic?

One of the roles of your preceptor is to introduce you to colleagues and multidisciplinary team members. Try to remember their names. Although this can be tricky at first some people have a knack for it and others do not; name badges and ward photo boards can help to jog your memory. It may also help if you get to know a bit about them, e.g. do they have children, what are their hobbies or interests? Having this information enables you to show an interest in colleagues; they appreciate it when you can ask about a particular event, e.g. a birthday party or their child's first day at school. It can also help you to understand why a colleague may, on occasion, not be their usual self. You also need to get to know your colleagues' strengths and weaknesses, e.g. who is good at dealing with aggressive or agitated patients, those with complex needs, or individuals with particular problems such as feeding. This can help you to get support in caring for your patients or to allocate staff when you start to coordinate the ward/area.

You need to develop an awareness of any cliques within the team and try to avoid being drawn into them. You need to tread a fine line between trying to get on with everyone and alienating colleagues. Keep an open mind to begin with and choose your loyalties carefully. You need to recognise that there are some people you will get on with less well than others and that work is the only thing you have in common with them. Accept this and work on being polite, courteous and professional to get you through these shifts.

One of the most useful things you can do as a new team member is to get to know your receptionist, if you have one. She/he is often a mine of useful information and has networks of contacts in other areas, potentially saving you frustrating phone calls to get things done.

Time management and prioritisation are hard skills to learn, and when done well, like much good nursing, are invisible. A useful starting point for ward-based staff is a sheet of paper that highlights your allocated patients and what needs doing when, for example, are there observations to be done, infusions to be read or observed and medicines to be given? This gives you an hour-by-hour breakdown of your workload in terms of tasks.

You then need to think about how to organise yourself. Do you have to go to the same patient three times in the space of 30 minutes to do different elements of care? It is tiring for both them and you and adds to the distance walked in a shift. Use your first few days in your new area to find out where things are kept and how they are ordered to ensure you can access all the equipment you need.

Think about how you can cluster care to make your contact more effective. As part of this, you need to be mindful of the workload of others and plan your own to take this into account. For example, it is no good presenting your colleague with a drug chart for intravenous antibiotics 5 minutes before they are due, and expect them to drop everything to administer them for you. This needs to be discussed at the start of the shift so that your colleague can incorporate it into his or her work.

If and when you are up to date with your work, you need to think how you are going to use your time. Try to avoid sitting at the desk making casual conversation with other staff; while this can be relaxing and useful for a short period of time, there are some other very useful things you can be doing. Offer to help out your colleagues, ensure that areas are stocked up and generally tidy: think how frustrating it is when someone else has used the last one of something and not replaced it. Is there one of your patients that would appreciate a little extra time? Even just combing a patient's hair or tidying their bed can help to develop a very therapeutic relationship. It is easy to get a label of being lazy, and very difficult to get rid of it once you have it – so it is best to avoid getting it in the first place.

For staff working in community settings, you will need to keep some sort of diary for planning your visits and to maintain your safety. Some patients may need to be seen at set times, for example because of their care needs or availability of other staff, whereas you have more flexibility with others.

Working with others

What does leadership and being in charge mean to you? These are not necessarily the same thing. Think about people you have worked with as a student. What were the leadership skills you admired in them? These are some of the things considered to be important:

- Fairness in workload allocation; this includes both the number and dependency of your patients.
- Being willing to help others out without being asked.
- Seeing when someone is struggling and being there to support them without taking over.
- Being able to take the lead when the situation demands it, e.g. in an emergency.

Issues to consider when in charge

- What is the skill mix of your team for that shift?
- How does this match the dependency levels of your patients, and do they have particular needs that only certain team members can meet?
- Take regular opportunities to update yourself on the state of the ward/ area/team, for example:
  - which patients are in or have come back from theatre?
  - who is being discharged?
  - are there any patients who have deteriorated or are causing concern?
  - Take steps to deal with issues as they arise, e.g. staff sickness – think about what impact this will have on subsequent shifts.
- Identify who is out there to help you: is there a duty manager or a bleepholder covering a floor or unit? They can often see the bigger picture, such as workloads in other areas, and help you reframe the

situation. However, it is important to demonstrate that you have tried to address the situation yourself. In some cases, you may just want to run a decision about something by them; on other occasions, you may need to utilise their experience and authority because you have exhausted your options. For example, if you cannot move anyone between shifts or find anyone who is off to do overtime, you need them to agree to arrange a bank nurse, move staff from another area or close beds.

How do I manage my time?
Claire Agnew

As nurses, we spend so much of our professional life looking after others that it is easy to forget to look after ourselves. From time management, having a social life, to looking after your career, I hope the following will help you through the day and point you in the right direction to achieving a happy and healthy career.

Time management

Ask yourself these questions:

- How many times have I not taken my break to get things done?
- How often do I get off work on time?
- How often do I get home and then phone work to pass on something I have forgotten?
- How long do I spend looking for things that I have lost or mislaid?

If your answer is 'sometimes' or 'frequently', then you need to develop some time management strategies to help you get through the day and feel you have achieved your goals at the end of it. Two important aspects of time management are: being more efficient (doing something right) and being more effective (doing the right thing).

Elements of time management include prioritising, putting things off and delegation.

Prioritising

- Write down everything that you have to do on a list and keep it with you all day.
- To help you see what needs to be done through the shift, divide the work into three main priorities and give them a ranking: 1 = urgent and important; 2 = important but less urgent; 3 = routine and low priority.
- As soon as you have completed a task, cross it off your list – nothing is more satisfying than seeing a list of tasks getting shorter.
- Be prepared to re-prioritise; a nurse's work is never static.
- Communicate with your team regularly throughout the shift so that you all know what is going on.
- Seek help and support from colleagues as soon as you feel that you are getting bogged down with work; never be afraid to ask.
- Only keep one list – any more and you will get confused as to where you are.

Putting things off

We put things off because:

- The task is overwhelming and we are frightened of failure.
- We have little or no information to start the task, are indecisive or are unsure of priorities.
- We cannot find things, or are too busy doing unimportant things.
- We may be stressed, ill or suffering from chronic fatigue.

Ways to move forward

- Tackle the worst or easiest task first.
- Break up the task into small manageable chunks.
- Do the parts of the task you feel you can do, then seek advice to help you complete it.

Delegation

An important aspect of time management for a qualified nurse is delegation. Reasons to delegate include:

- It frees more time for the jobs only you can do.
- It allows others to learn new tasks.
- It encourages motivation to become a more useful member of the team.
- The job may be done better by someone else.

Why we do not delegate:

- We feel we can do the job better.
- We do the job quicker.
- We enjoy doing the job.
- It is a habit.
- We fear letting go as someone else may do the task better.

The best ways to delegate:

- Choose the person most suitable for the job.
- Ensure that they are capable of doing the task.
- Explain the job and ask them if they foresee any problems.
- Leave them to get on with it.
- Ask them how they got on and help them deal with any unresolved issues.

(Hindle, 1998; Martin, 2000)

How do I get to grips with working unsocial hours?

Claire Agnew

Requesting off duty

We all deserve a life outside work. How often is it said that the off-duty folder rules our lives? Working with newly qualified nurses, I am never surprised that they quite often forget to book annual leave or fill out extra duty forms – this is easily done when you are getting to grips with a new job. The average person has many things to juggle throughout the day – work, partners, family, friends and further study – yet it is still important to look after your own health and wellbeing.

Points to remember when making off-duty requests:

- Be fair – your team members would like to have a life as well.
- Plan ahead – there is no point expecting to get the days off you want if you do not go to book them until the week before.
- Remember, most off duty is planned 6–8 weeks ahead.
- Do not go for 4 months without a holiday or you will be too burnt out to enjoy it.
- Space your annual leave evenly throughout the year.
- Follow any local guidelines set for leave requests or self-rostering, such as allowing only certain numbers of staff off at any one time or booking the weekend off before annual leave.

Special duty payments

Nursing is a 24-hour, 7 day a week profession; working nights, weekends and bank holidays are all part of the job. However, most nurses get some financial reward for working these 'unsocial hours', which is claimed for by filling in the appropriate forms from your place of work. It is your responsibility to fill out any paperwork related to special duty payments, and to ensure that you get the applicable shifts signed for on the days you work. You may be asked to sign forms for other staff; if you do, it is your responsibility to be certain that they worked the hours written on the form.

Maintaining a social life while doing shift work

Work should stay at work, and home should stay at home, but how easy is this to achieve? The important thing to remember is that it is all about maintaining a balance. Does working 12-hour shifts, doing three nights, having two days off and back on an early shift sound like a nightmare?

Welcome to the world of nursing and 24-hour care. Shift work can be difficult to get used to and it is important that you are fit to function when on duty. Gone are the days when, as a student, you could have a late night out and be able to function on the early shift the next day; you are now an accountable practitioner and need to be able to function as one.

On the other hand, if you are getting many nine to 10 day stretches and a quick turn around from days to nights, and then back to days, you need to discuss this with your preceptor, mentor, ward sister or line manager. Becoming tired and stressed through shift work could affect your patient care – it is important to recognise this. You need to do something positive about it and seek out support mechanisms.

What should I expect from clinical supervision?

Claire Agnew

Clinical supervision is a process that promotes personal and professional development within a supportive relationship. It aims to promote high clinical standards and develop professional expertise by supporting staff and promoting an ethos of openness and honesty in the practice setting, and helps to develop personal awareness of strengths and weaknesses (Fowler, 1999; Wheeler, 2001; McSherry et al, 2002).

Sounds wonderful, but does it happen in practice? In my experience, although there are some areas that fully support clinical supervision, it is something that is often suggested after the nurse has experienced a distressing incident, and not something that is ingrained in practice. As nurses working in a stressful profession, we need to look after ourselves: clinical supervision provides an opportunity to discuss clinical issues and professional practice in a secure environment with someone with whom you feel comfortable and with whom you can work towards solutions.

As you are a qualified nurse, your managers have a duty to provide clinical supervision if you request it (Fowler, 1999). Do not be afraid to ask for clinical supervision – it is not a sign of weakness. Most examples of clinical supervision are based on local arrangements that are dependent of the needs of the staff. It would not be unrealistic to expect a one-to-one meeting of about an hour once a month with your clinical supervisor. Between meetings you would be expected to reflect upon your practice and bring to the meeting any concerns that you have.

How do I deal with experienced healthcare assistants?
Karen Jackson

You may feel quite inadequate or threatened if you are responsible for supervising some very experienced staff, such as qualified nurses or healthcare assistants. Healthcare assistants often have considerable experience and are very familiar with the ward routine. Make sure that you treat everyone with equal respect. If you gain people's respect, they will work with you and for you. Work hard and enthusiastically and you will find that staff will follow your lead. Do not be frightened or embarrassed to ask people's opinions and advice.

Healthcare assistants often spend more time with a patient than you do, so make sure you ask them how they think Mrs Smith is coping with her colostomy, anxiety, new medication or whatever, and value their feedback. Make sure you understand how healthcare assistants fit into the team. Do they have allocated patients overseen by a trained nurse or do they help out generally, such as by assisting with personal hygiene? You need to agree with them who is doing what and when on a shift. There is little point in them bathing a patient when you have just spent 30 minutes doing their wound dressing.

Do not be afraid to ask others within the team to help you out but recognise that learning to delegate is hard. It is easy to run yourself ragged trying to do everything for all your patients because you want to be seen as a good nurse who can cope. It may sound obvious, but how you ask makes a difference. You do not want to come over as either lazy or bossy. A comment often heard from healthcare assistants about newly qualified nurses is that they would have been happy to help if only they had been asked.

The knowledge and experience of healthcare assistants varies considerably and you should not assume that a person is competent to undertake a certain duty simply because they have worked in that area for two years. You may feel uncomfortable asking an experienced healthcare assistant, who may be quite a bit older than you, if they know how to do something. However, you are the accountable practitioner and you are responsible for ensuring that the person you are asking to do something has the necessary skills and knowledge to undertake it safely. They are, in turn, responsible for recognising their limitations and not taking on aspects of care that they are not competent to perform. You need to be aware of what individuals can or cannot do, and your trust's policy in assessing competence.

What am I meant to do on a ward round?

Karen Jackson

Ward rounds vary in style and duration, and so the contribution of the nurse varies. However, a key element of the role is to represent the patients' interests, either by enabling them to make their needs known or to do so yourself where they are unwilling or unable. You need to be clear that it is their view that is being articulated, and not your perception of what you think they want or need.

If the round takes place on a ward, position yourself so that you are with your patients and not buried three deep in a crowd of medical students. Ensure that all relevant documentation is available and up to date. You may not know the observations for all the patients on the ward, but can refer to the relevant charts.

Make sure that any equipment needed is available and working. This will make you appear efficient and you will not waste time looking for things, by which time the round has moved on and you have missed your opportunity to raise your concerns about a particular patient. Ensure that you understand any changes to treatment plans. If your area uses a ward round book, keep this up to date or keep your own notes so that changes can be communicated to colleagues, and documentation/plans of care amended accordingly. Again, you need to understand how the team works. For example, are request cards and prescriptions written as the round progresses or are they all done at the end?

Be aware of infection control issues, ensure items such as gloves and aprons are available and used appropriately, and remind medical staff to wash their hands between patients. Ensure that items such as stethoscopes are appropriately decontaminated.

What do I need to know about the research process?
Karen Jackson

The need for evidence-based practice underpins modern healthcare provision and links closely with the Clinical Governance agenda. Thompson and Learmouth (2002) suggest that an evidence-based decision has four elements:

- Evidence from research.
- Clinical experience.
- Available resources.
- Patient preference.

Remember that just as we have access to a wide range of information, so do our service users. Glen and Cox (2006) comment that nurses have to develop a facilitative role in helping individuals evaluate the information they have read.

There has probably never been so much research taking place, so why does it seem that nursing continues ritualistic practice, with learning the ward routine crucial to your survival as a new staff nurse? How can you ensure that your practice is evidence based without alienating your colleagues? This raises a number of questions:

- Is there evidence to support what we do and how good is it?
- Do workload pressures enable us to critically evaluate our practice?
- Are there leaders for change?
- Can we define good nursing care; are all the elements measurable?

On a day-to-day basis, policies and guidelines provide a fertile area for evidence-based practice and it should be possible to identify the rationale on which any recommendations have been made. Find out when these were last updated. If you have an interest in a particular area, you may be able to get involved in work relating to it which in turn will support your ongoing continuing professional development and achievement of your Knowledge and Skills Framework (KSF) competencies.

You need to be critical about ideas you have read about before considering implementing them in your area. Newman and Roberts (2002) identify three elements within this:

- Is the quality of the study good enough to use the results?
- Are the findings applicable in my setting?
- What do the results mean for my patients?

Consider how you can utilise opportunities such as ward meetings to introduce new ideas and consider how they might be implemented. However, you need to remember that not everyone will be so keen. It may well have been tried before and not worked; who can you persuade to give it another go or do you need to consider something else?

Snowball (1999) identified five key questions to be asked when looking at research:

- What type of question is being asked?
- What sort of information would provide evidence to answer this type of question?
- What type of study would provide such information?
- What types of information resources would give access to these studies?
- How do we get the best out of resources?

Most research texts include guidelines on how to critique research. The main areas you need to consider are:

- *Comprehension*: Is the topic under investigation clearly identified? Is there a research question and theoretical framework? Are hypotheses to be tested stated where applicable?
- *Comparison and analysis*: How has the literature review been done? Is the selection of methodology and methods appropriate, with evidence of the decision-making process, including issues of rigour such as reliability and validity? How have the data been collected and analysed? Have ethical issues been addressed? What limitations to the study are identified?
- *Evaluation*: Have results been interpreted appropriately, e.g. use of statistical tests or the categorisation of qualitative data? Is the interpretation of the results consistent with the findings, and can claims be justified?

What implications for practice are identified?

Most research texts will offer more detailed guidance regarding these issues as different questions need to be asked depending on the methodology chosen, i.e. the underpinning philosophy, which broadly translates into either quantitative or qualitative, which in turn influences the method used.

Working in a research role

If you want to undertake research in your area, you will need to think this through very carefully. Factors to consider are:

- Whose cooperation will you need to carry out the project and change practice?
- What ethical considerations are there?
- Will you receive support in terms of time and administrative support to undertake the work?

Badly done research will do nothing to enhance your reputation. It may be appropriate at this stage in your career to identify the opportunities that exist within your directorate or trust for promoting research if this is something you are interested in. Many trusts have a research and development directorate, which may be able to offer advice and support or you may be able to make links with a local university. Think about setting up an interest group with like-minded colleagues to share ideas and good practice. For example, children's nurses have access to a network of local groups known as Research in Child Health (RiCH) via the Royal College of Nursing (RCN).

How can we begin to evaluate practice?

John Fowler

If we are going to evaluate practice developments we then need to ask what exactly are we going to evaluate? Is it our views as practitioners, the clients' views, the managers' views, patient outcomes, morality rate? One of the first rules of evaluation is to be very clear about what it is you want to evaluate. You will need to acknowledge that you probably will not be able to evaluate everything. You will also need to recognise that, while you are evaluating one or two areas probably from one perspective, then the practice development may be having other effects that you may or may not recognise. Thus what you will be finding is probably at best a partial evaluation and you must avoid the danger of making claims that cannot be substantiated by your evaluation procedure. Consider the following example regarding the evaluation of hand washing techniques following the use of the toilet by qualified nurses. Review the examples of how this may be done:

- The nurse in charge of the ward carries out interviews with all her staff regarding their habits.
- The nurse in charge describes what she believes to be the standard habits based upon her knowledge of her staff.
- The nurse in charge gives each nurse a questionnaire to fill in and return in person to her after 20 minutes.
- An independent researcher carries out interviews with the staff.
- An independent researcher conducts an anonymous questionnaire.
- A reporter from the local paper asks nurses about their habits.
- An independent researcher takes a seat in the toilets and openly observes people's hand washing habits.
- A hidden camera is placed in the toilets (above the wash basins) and is monitored secretly from another location.

Such is the complexity of human behaviour that I would suggest that the only valid evaluation would be the last. It would be interesting to see if ethical permission could be gained for such a study, I doubt it. Absurd as the example is, how many 'evaluations' of clinical practice have you seen published that are based on any of the first seven examples? Sadly, too many. If we are going to evaluate practice we firstly have to be focused on what it is we are trying to evaluate. We must then measure what can be measured and having measured one thing – 'A' – not begin to imply that we have really measured 'B', which is something completely different.

There is considerable difficulty in evaluating areas that involve multiple factors. The simplest form of evaluation can occur when a single factor has a single effect. An example of this might be a pharmacological agent that has been developed to act on a specific receptor, which leads to a reduction in blood pressure. However, even with this example, it is rare for one drug to have a single effect. Although there are some aspects of nursing and healthcare that might be considered in this single cause and effect way, the majority of healthcare is far more complex and multi-factorial.

Consider the factors affecting how patients feel about being admitted to hospital:

- Have they been on a waiting list for a long time?
- Have they had a previous admission cancelled?
- Have they been in pain?
- Is this an emergency admission?
- Is the condition life threatening?
- Is it embarrassing?
- Does it involve a moral dilemma?
- How did they arrive at the hospital?
- Have they come with someone?
- Could they park the car?
- Have they left a dependent relative at home?

and so on.

What about nurses admitting patients:

- Is this their sixth day on duty?
- Are they due off duty in 10 minutes but someone asked them to admit this patient before they leave?
- Were they expecting the admission?
- Have they had a chance to read the notes and familiarise themselves with the patient's background?
- Have they just broken up with their partner?
- Has the ward sister just told them off?
- Have they just been promoted?
- Are they the same age, ethnic background, gender as the patient?

These are just a few of the factors that will influence the way a patient feels about being admitted to hospital. Some of the factors are going to be more important for all patients, e.g. the life-threatening nature of the condition, but others may affect only a few, and others, although affecting the majority of patients, may not feel important. Equally, most of nursing and related healthcare involves a similar web of complex factors, which are often taken for granted, particularly when nurses are exposed to them every day. If we then inject a new factor into the admission of a patient, e.g. an admission room or an admission nurse or a reserved car space, how can we tell whether is it this new factor that is improving the quality of the admission and not a change in one or a number of the other ones, of which we are unaware?

Evaluation of some of the most fundamental roles of healthcare workers is an enormously difficult task. It is like trying to unweave a tapestry to see why it creates a picture. You need to be able to see each thread in relation to the one next to it and the effect that changing the colour of one tread will have on others. Although the picture may look quite simple to start with, once you begin to take it to pieces, you realise how complicated the interactions are. The addition of one or two extra threads in certain places may have little obvious impact but may change the overall picture completely.

What is the best method of evaluation?

There is not one method of evaluation that is the best. However there are more appropriate methods depending on the nature of the situation being evaluated. Different methods are also more robust in terms of their ability to predict similar outcomes in future events.

Randomised controlled trials (RCTs)

This often referred to as the 'gold standard' of evaluation (Shepperd et al, 1997). An RCT is a longitudinal study in which participants are randomly selected into two groups. One group is given the 'treatment' that is being studied and the other group, the control group, is given nothing. Comparisons are then made between the treatment group and the control group. There are various levels of sophistication of RCTs using double or triple blind approaches, in which the practitioners and researchers are not aware of which group the patient is in, and whether one patient is receiving the 'treatment' or a placebo. If the RCT is well designed with the control and treatment group being as similar as possible with all possible bias being eliminated, and the 'treatment' is a single or easily identified variable and the outcomes objectively measurable, then the evaluative and predictive power of the RCT cannot be bettered. RCTs are used predominantly with pharmacological treatments although there are a few examples of RCTs being used in surgery and other areas (Shepperd et al, 1997).

Before and after studies

Before and after studies (Polit and Hungler, 1995) are another form of longitudinal study in which baseline measurements are made prior to the introduction of a treatment and then similar measurements are made following the introduction. Comparisons are then made between the before and after measurement and conclusions drawn. The difficulty with before and after studies is that other variables apart from the treatment may be introduced over the time period. A number of medical conditions improve on their own over a period of time with no external treatment. If we were to conduct a before and after study on patients with back pain and the treatment was to put a plaster on their back for four weeks, then we would probably find that a significant number of patients would say that their pain had subsided during the study. We might then claim that our treatment, the plaster, worked. It would not be difficult to exchange the plaster for a slightly more exotic treatment, which could then be marketed and sold. Another before and after study might be to measure staff morale before and after the introduction of new management system, but again the two measurements can be contaminated by a number of other variables. Before and after studies are useful and will often be used to evaluate a new system of healthcare or approach to nursing.

Provided the results and conclusions are presented within the context of other variables that may have had an influence, then they can be useful in giving general direction and views on what effect the 'treatment' had. However they cannot be used in the same way as a well-designed RCT.

Case studies

Case studies (Bowling, 1997) focus on a single person or example of what is being studied. They are another example of a longitudinal study that follows a person over a period of time. They may incorporate regular measurements or interviews with the subject. Case studies tend to take a more holistic view of the situation, trying to acknowledge and possibly prioritise the variety of interacting variables that may have affected the person or situation. A case study could take place on a single patient or it could be a case study looking at an outpatient department or a medical ward. The results and conclusions from a case study approach can be used to give new and more holistic insights into what is happening in a particular situation. What might have been true for the person in the case study might also be relevant to others. What worked in one outpatients or one ward might be appropriate in another similar area. However, the emphasis must be on the words 'might be relevant' to other similar situations.

Case studies are particularly useful in giving a holistic picture to an event and also in their ability to identify important variables that may have a significant influence on a situation. Their strength, which is also their weakness, is that they allow human judgement to interact with a complex multi-variable situation, appreciating the holistic nature of the event as well as identifying possible quirks that may be influencing the situation.

Surveys

Surveys (Bowling, 1997) take a snap shot of a situation, often using questionnaires or interviews. Surveys usually begin by identifying a particular group of the population, e.g. patients attending a particular outpatient department, children with asthma, diabetic specialist nurses, etc. Using appropriate sampling techniques a proportion of that group is identified. The sample group is then asked certain questions, usually via a questionnaire or sometimes face-to-face. Alternatively, the survey may involve some form of test, observation or investigation, e.g. the blood pressure or body weight of the sample group. Provided the sample group has been randomly selected from the population, then the results from the sample can be generalised back to the population. Surveys vary considerable in quality depending upon the degree of randomisation of the sample, design of the questionnaire, response rate, and analysis of the results. They are particularly useful in gaining a general view of a particular group of the population, often being used to gain patient or staff satisfaction views.

Working in practice

If you are going to invest considerable time, energy and resources into developing your practice, then it makes sense that you should also evaluate that practice. The form of evaluation needs to be included in the initial planning stage.

You may want to include a before and after study or conduct a baseline measure of patient satisfaction. Many of these measurements will be lost once the practice development has started, and if you only begin to consider evaluation once the development is in progress you will find it very difficult to carry out any form of comparative study. Therefore, the first important point in evaluation is to include it in the original planning stage of the development. If at all possible include in this planning stage a person who has a specific remit to oversee the evaluation. If you are coming from a largely clinical background then you may want to invite a research officer or university member to take on this role. The next point is to be as focused as possible in identifying the variable involved in the practice development and the outcomes expected. What is it you want to do and what are you going to measure to see if this has occurred? It is very tempting with a development to jump straight in and get so involved with running it that you lose track of the wider issues. It is here that a practice development team can give direction, support and feedback regarding the implementation and evaluation of the development. This may involve additional resources, which may be available from within the trust or from outside agencies. A practice development team will be in a far stronger position to access additional resources than someone working in isolation. Selection procedures for any additional funding, although time-consuming, are likely to focus your thoughts on both the form of practice development and the style of evaluation.

If your practice development is already under way and you did not incorporate an evaluation strategy from the start, then you can still undertake some form of evaluation. This may be a survey of satisfaction or a measure of patient throughput or waiting times, etc. Some of these measures may be comparable to similar national statistics. Even at this stage you would be well advised to engage an independent person to act as evaluator. In any evaluation the person implementing the development is likely to be seen as being biased, even if the evaluation was objectively undertaken.

Having undertaken some innovative form of practice development, and hopefully having undertaken some form of evaluation of the development, you must then publish your results. Again there are benefits here of a team approach. If you have implemented and evaluated the practice development yourself, you will probably have run out of energy by the time you have some results worth publishing. If you have worked as part of a team, with different people having responsibility for different aspects of the development, then when you come to publication the team will act as a motivator.

Publication in appropriate journals and sharing of experiences at conferences are both a little daunting if you work alone and have not experienced this form of presentation before. Working within a team which incorporates people with different skills and experiences can help take a development from planning through implementation and evaluation to publication of results.

What issues are involved in obtaining consent?
Karen Jackson

- What do we mean by consent?
- What do people need to consent to?
- Who can give consent for children, young people and adults?
- When can we proceed without consent?

We tend to think of consent as the signing of forms for surgery and other procedures, but consent is generally obtained for most of what we do and is an ongoing process. Some of this is what is known as implied consent. For example, when we ask patients if we can record their blood pressure, they put their arm out to enable us to apply the cuff. In this situation it is likely that the patient is familiar with what is going to happen and it is accepted that this is part of the routine.

With regard to a blood test, for example, we may need to give a little more information, such as where the blood will be taken from, how much will be taken, who will take it and what tests will be carried out on it. Here, the individual agreeing to the sample being taken would imply consent. Consent forms are generally used for procedures that involve something more invasive, which might be done under sedation or an anaesthetic. The process involves an opportunity to weigh up the risks and benefits of having the procedure, what it involves, other options and any implications of not having the treatment.

Having a signed form is a record of when discussions took place, but not proof of consent. It is not uncommon to find that your patient still has unanswered questions, despite having signed the form, and you will need to be proactive in ensuring that these are answered by an appropriate individual. It may be useful to help patients to identify specific questions that they have and explore the use of alternatives, such as diagrams, to enable understanding. The issues of taking samples during surgery and the disposal of body parts were highlighted by events at Alder Hey Children's Hospital (Redfern Report, www.rlcinquiry.org.uk/download/index.htm). The consent process therefore needs to ensure that individuals are aware of why samples are being taken. Usually this is to enable further treatment, such as samples for biopsy, but it may also be for research purposes. Consent issues link to the clinical governance agenda. For example, elements of the patient-focus domain in Standards for Better Health (Department of Health, 2004) look at having consent systems in place, treatment with care and respect, and access to services in terms of treatment, care and aftercare.

With regard to who can give consent, a number of aspects need to be considered.

Children under 16

For children under 16 years of age, consent can be given by someone with parental responsibility. Parental responsibility is automatically held by mothers and married parents including marriage following conception or birth. For unmarried fathers, the situation is different:

- Where the child is born before 1 December 2003, parental responsibility order can be obtained or an agreement registered with the court.
- For those born after this date, the previous options can be used but in addition, it can be obtained by joint registration of the birth.

Parental responsibility may be shared in certain circumstances, e.g. the child in care, which may involve the local authority and other family members.

Children should be involved in the consent process; this raises the concept of 'Gillick' competence, where an assessment is made of whether there is sufficient understanding, intelligence and maturity to comprehend what is proposed. The achievement of competence depends both on the child and the severity or complexity of the treatment (Griffith and Tengnah, 2008). Alderson (1993) notes that quite young children can give consent if they are involved in the process, particularly in the case of chronic illness, although they may still want their parents to give consent. Where the child cannot give consent it is useful to consider what elements of the process they can be involved in, e.g. having medication from an oral syringe or spoon, or what toy will accompany them to theatre. The concept of 'Gillick' competence also applies to parents under the age of 16, and they can give consent for their child if they are assessed as competent.

Young people aged 16 or 17 years

This age group are presumed in law to be competent under the Family Law Reform Act (1969), and can therefore give their own consent although there are limitations to this. It may be necessary to consider whether the family needs to be involved in the process and agreement sought on this. Young people with learning difficulties may be able to give consent if information is presented in an appropriate way, but the person with parental responsibility can give consent if needed.

Adults

Adults themselves are the only ones who can give consent for procedures involving them although in an emergency situation it is lawful to provide immediate and necessary treatment without consent. Where it becomes apparent that additional procedures are needed during a course of treatment, it is necessary to obtain further consent unless such a delay would be detrimental to an individual's life or health.

The new Mental Capacity Act (2005) provides guidance in the assessment of whether adults can make an informed decision. It has five key principles as follows:

- Presumption of capacity unless proven otherwise.
- Support for individuals to make decisions; the format in which information is presented and alternatives to enable understanding must be considered.
- Unwise decisions may not indicate a lack of capacity.
- Best interests, including consideration of previous requests and expressed beliefs; who else needs to be involved in the consultation.
- Least restrictive option in terms of individuals' rights and freedom of action.

Where an individual has been shown to lack capacity, the Act makes a number of provisions to compensate for that and to support the consent process.

The use of interpreters in obtaining consent needs to be considered. Implications for confidentiality must be taken into account. This is particularly pertinent where the individual and interpreter both come from the same community, as they may be known to each other and the patient may be reluctant to discuss personal matters with them.

The use of family members also raises issues. Children, for example, may not understand the information given and be unable to translate it accurately. Other adults may only interpret selective information on the basis of what they think the person needs to know. Both situations mean that the individual concerned cannot make an informed decision. Remember that some things may be translated literally and the meaning lost. Some years ago, I was involved in putting together advice leaflets on HIV and AIDS. It became apparent that in one of the leaflets, anal sex had been translated as sex via the back door – not quite what was meant! At the same time, it is necessary to be sensitive to the needs of the individual and family, and in some situations the advice of senior members of the community may be sought when making a decision.

What is involved in professional development?
Claire Agnew

As nurses, we are accountable for maintaining a high standard of professional practice. Healthcare provision is an environment of constant change and it is vital that all nurses are able to keep up with this. Lifelong learning is a concept that gets bandied around in official-sounding documents, but within nursing it is grounded in our professional development: once you start learning, you cannot stop (Nursing and Midwifery Council, 2002).

Post-registration education and practice (PREP) is a set of Nursing and Midwifery Council (NMC) standards and guidelines that enable you to demonstrate that you are keeping up to date with developments in professional practice and to embrace the concepts of lifelong learning. They include keeping a personal professional profile (see Box) and completing a certain amount of hours on continuing professional development.

What a professional profile will do for you

- Help you assess your current standards of practice
- Develop your analytical skills
- Review and evaluate past experience
- Demonstrate experiential learning
- Assist with job or course applications

The PREP Handbook is a comprehensive guide to meeting the standards set. The latest revision was published by the NMC in 2004, and is available free of charge through the organisation's website (www.nmc-uk.org). I recommend obtaining this for detailed information on PREP, but here are some of the issues covered:

- PREP does not have to cost you any money.
- There is no such thing as an approved PREP continuing professional development activity.
- You do not need to collect points or certificates.
- There is no approved format for the personal professional profile.
- PREP must be relevant to the work you are doing or plan to do.
- PREP must help you provide the highest possible standards of care for your patients.

Many employers are now recognising the importance of staff development, and that by investing in this they are developing a competent, motivated and committed workforce. One way of achieving this is through appraisal or individual performance reviews (Wheeler, 2001). This provides you with the chance to sit down with your manager and plan your career; it does not matter if your career aspirations are just surviving your night shift – the important thing is that you get the opportunity to discuss your strengths and weaknesses and develop an action plan for achieving your goals. In my experience, new nurses tend to focus on the acquisition of clinical skills, getting their intravenous (IV) and cannulation certificate, and life support skills. However, it is important not to overlook your development in areas such as assertiveness, team working and time management skills.

Planning your professional development should include:

- A review of your competence.
- Setting your learning objectives.
- Developing an action plan.
- Implementing an action plan.
- Evaluation of what happened.
- Record of your study time and learning outcomes.

Strengths
• *Professional manner*
• *Easy to get on with*
• *Friendly, but assertive*

Strengths
- *Professional manner*
- *Easy to get on with*
- *Friendly, but assertive*

Weaknesses
- *Can't say no*
- *Leave things until the last minute*
- *Clinical skills*

Opportunities
- *Secondment*
- *Shadowing other staff*
- *Being a mentor*

Threats
- *Shortage of staff*
- *Keeping motivated*
- *Over-committing myself*

Name	Signature	Date
Job title	Manager	Review date
Career aspirations / development pathway		

Figure 5.1. Example of a SWOT analysis.

You can undertake a SWOT analysis to help identify your strengths, weaknesses, opportunities and threats. *Figure 5.1* shows an example of this. A framework for developing a personal professional development plan is shown in *Figure 5.2*.

Name	Signature	Date
Job title	Manager	Review date
Career aspirations / development pathway		
Personal learning objective	Action agreed	Timescales: Complete?:

Figure 5.2. Personal development plan.

How can I develop my professional practice?
John Fowler

There are many opportunities for professional development. However, those available to you at any one time will vary depending upon:

- Your vision for your career pathway.
- Your strengths and weaknesses.
- The amount of additional time you are willing and able to invest in your development.
- The culture of the area in which you work.

Some opportunities will be given to you; others may be available, but you will have to take an active part in seeking and taking them; others you will have to seek out and seize.

The development of professional practice cannot happen as an isolated event. It is part of a process of clinical experience, deepening of underpinning knowledge and exploration and development of your interpersonal skills.

Potential opportunities are listed below. Some will be available to you now, and others may become available to you over the next few years.

- *Clinical experience*
  - Make sure you build up an in-depth knowledge of the specialty in which you work. This includes the practice and skills of that area, and the underpinning physiological, psychological and pharmacological knowledge of the specialty and any legal and professional issues that are relevant.
  - Consider working in a different clinical specialty and broadening your clinical experience. Some clinical managers will safeguard your E grade if you change specialties by providing you with a fast-track in-service development programme for a new specialty. Be prepared to ask and negotiate these sorts of conditions when planning your development.
  - Consider working in a different hospital, a different part of the country or working abroad. Obviously this option is not available to everyone and will depend upon your personal and social circumstances.
  - Length of experience is not the same as breadth and depth of experience. If you are spending 5 or 10 years in one clinical area, make sure that you become the most knowledgeable and skilled person in that specialty. Beware of becoming someone who has one year's experience 10 times.
- *Preceptorship and clinical supervision*: One of the most effective ways of making sure that you learn and develop from your clinical experience is

to obtain help and advice from someone more experienced than yourself. Clinical supervision helps you to focus on specific events and examine them in a reflective and developmental way. It is your right to have clinical supervision; this is often difficult to organise in busy clinical areas, but if you persevere it will happen and will be useful.

- *Study days and in-service training*: These are study days or short courses concerned with helping you to work in your specialty. They may involve certain mandatory courses, such as moving and handling or food hygiene, or they may be more specific to your clinical area, such as IV medication and child protection procedures. Take the opportunity not only to attend these days but also to help in their administration or, if appropriate, to lead them.

- *Short courses and open learning programmes*: There are a number of useful learning packs produced by a variety of people or institutions. For example, there may be a locally produced learning pack on hip replacements or interpreting ECGs, or a more professional pack on using spreadsheets or health education, or *Nursing Times* or *Nursing* learning packs.

- *Standard professional development series*. These courses are not usually assessed by a college or university, but are very useful in helping you to develop specific skills and knowledge that are relevant to your needs and clinical area.

- *Validated programmes*: These are usually Diplomas of Higher Education or Bachelors or Masters degrees. They will involve several years of part-time study, so make sure you pick the right course for you.

- *Secondment*: Occasionally, opportunities arise for a member of staff to be seconded to undertake a specific role away from her/his normal working environment. This may be within your own trust, such as transferring to another ward to cover maternity leave or to help set up a new unit. Other opportunities may include secondment to another organisation to help develop, audit or teach. These are very useful opportunities as they expose you to different ways of working and different structures for a limited period of time while maintaining the security of your employment in your original base area.

- *Research*: This may be a rather frightening option for a number of staff. However, there are many different levels at which you can be involved in research. At the simplest stage it can involve simply becoming aware of any research that is being undertaken in your area or trust. Once you have found out what is happening, try to get involved, initially perhaps by helping out with tasks such as collecting data, sorting or photocopying. Just being involved in the research process with experienced researchers will increase your knowledge and help you to make useful contacts.

What sort of post-registration course should I do?
Nigel Goodrich and John Fowler

As discussed in the previous section, there are a number of important study days that a newly qualified nurse should undertake. These are usually organised locally, either by the unit training officer or more centrally by your employing trust or hospital. Some of these are mandatory; others are specific to the clinical area in which you are working. These study days involve particular skills or procedures that enable you to work effectively in your area. They may be concerned with IV therapy, administering medications, moving and handling, infection control, etc. These are important and are usually undertaken in the first year after qualifying. As part of your preceptorship you should have identified your 'learning needs' and discussed them with a more senior member of staff. This should continue with an annual review of your performance and any training that you require – your individual performance review (IPR).

The next significant development that you should be contemplating is the mentorship course. You may already have been assisting with the support and teaching of students; however, before you can take full responsibility for overseeing a student on a placement you will need to undertake an NMC accredited mentorship course. Your local university will almost certainly run mentorship courses and your application and place on the course is usually coordinated by your line manager in conjunction with a trust training officer. Most managers would expect all E grades to have undertaken, or be in the process of completing, the mentorship course, and be taking an active part in mentoring students.

Following a mentorship course, there are no specific 'rules' as to what, if any, further courses you should undertake. It is important that you seek advice before investing considerable amounts of time, energy and possibly money into further study. Some clinical areas have traditionally provided and expected staff to undergo further studies in order for them to work effectively, e.g. intensive care units, accident and emergency units, and orthopaedics, whereas other areas, such as medicine and surgery, have tended to expect staff to develop their skills and knowledge based on experience.

It is important for you to find out what is currently valued in the area in which you wish to specialise. This can be part of your IPR or clinical supervision sessions.

A common national standard is the NMC's Specialist Practitioner Award. This is a post-registration award validated by the organisation, which is usually based on degree studies in an area or specialty. The Specialist Practitioner Programme prepares staff to exercise high levels of judgement and clinical decision making and is based on four key areas (United Kingdom Central Council for Nursing, Midwifery and Health Visiting, 1994):

- Specialist clinical practice.
- Care and programme management.
- Clinical practice leadership.
- Clinical practice development.

The majority of universities that provide undergraduate nurse training will also have a post-registration degree that is part of the NMC Specialist Practitioner Award. Most universities will have a course that enables nurses who have undertaken a pre-registration diploma of nursing to continue with degree studies and complete a degree that incorporates a NMC Specialist Practitioner Award.

Building on your Diploma in Nursing, this can usually be completed part time in two years and will normally incorporate a subspecialty such as critical care nursing, mental health nursing or surgical nursing. Nurses who have undertaken a pre-registration degree in nursing should also aim to complete a NMC Specialist Practitioner Award. Some universities may offer this as part of a Master's programme, but others may only offer it at first-degree level.

Once nurses have achieved the following they can start applying for F grade or equivalent posts.

- Gained appropriate experience, usually a minimum of three years.
- Completed the mentorship course and is experienced in mentoring.
- Normally completed a degree that incorporates a specialist area of nursing practice.

Nurses who wish to continue with their career may contemplate such posts as nurse specialist, practice development nurse or nurse lecturer, but would normally need two further years of experience that includes leadership and management experience and have commenced or completed an appropriate Master's degree.

It is quite probable that future nurse consultants will not only have national reputations of clinical excellence and research, but also be engaged in or have completed doctorate degree studies.

If all this seems a bit daunting and remote from patient care, do not despair. The majority of post-registration nursing courses are designed to enhance and develop client/patient care. Not all nurses need to be undertaking post-registration degrees; however, if you want to take a key role in developing client/patient care, then you need to consider how you will acquire the appropriate underpinning skills, knowledge and attitudes required to develop professional practice.

What are CAT points and APAs?
John Fowler

The majority of university degrees are structured into modules of study that are given a certain amount of points or credits. A degree is made up of a fixed quota of credits within certain subject areas. The majority of universities have agreed a set formula that allows a certain amount of transferability between different universities. Some combination of the following terminology is usually used:

- Year one certificate level 4 (this used to be called level 1).
- Year two diploma level 5 (this used to be called level 2).
- Year three degree level 6 (this used to be called level 3).

Each year or level is made up of 120 credits. A full honours degree is made up of 120 credits at level 4, 120 credits at level 5, plus 120 credits at level 6, giving a total of 360 credits. Universities allocate different amounts of credits to modules of study, but the total amount will still add up to 120 for each level.

Thus some universities may structure their courses as 10 modules of 12 credits each, another may have eight modules of 15 credits each and others may use a combination of 15-, 30- and 60-credit modules within their courses. The important fact is that each year or level totals 120 credits.

Courses that are run on a part-time basis have the same structure consisting of level 4, level 5 and level 6, but level 4 may take place over two years rather than one year as in the traditional full-time structure. Pre-registration diploma courses contain the academic content of level 4 and level 5 studies, but are taught over a three-year period. This is due to the fact that nurses will not only qualify with a diploma in higher education in nursing, but also with a registered nurse professional qualification. There is currently a move to take all pre-registration nursing courses to full degree qualification, thus students will complete a total of 360 credits at levels 4, 5 and 6.

A number of nurses will undertake a short course or module at a university, which, although not a full degree, will normally attract credits, e.g. 30 level 5 credits or 30 level 6 credits. These are very useful and not only demonstrate continuing professional development but also the ability to study at level 6. However, simply collecting 360 credits will not necessarily be all that is required to complete a degree. A diploma or degree is made up of specific subjects, not simply the accumulation of the required number of points. Thus a degree in nursing is normally made up of modules on: research, leadership, teaching, nursing practice, physiology, psychology, and sociology – all applied to healthcare. Simply collecting 360 credits that are only concerned with one, two or three of these subjects will not demonstrate that you have covered the syllabus of a nursing degree.

There are some specific terms associated with credits and how they can be used in a flexible way sometimes in different universities:

- *Degree*: Only a university can award a degree (360 credits).
- *Diploma of Higher Education*: Only a university can award a Diploma of Higher Education (DipHE – 240 credits).
- *Diploma*: Anyone can issue a diploma, provided that it does not say Diploma of Higher Education. So beware of paying a lot of money for a diploma that you may see advertised. The diploma may also refer to learning points or professional points – beware, these are not higher education points as awarded by a university. This is not to say that these diplomas are not worth anything; often they may provide useful information and sometimes they are validated by a professional body, but they will not count towards your degree.
- *Certificate of Higher Education*: This is awarded by a university (CertHE – 120 credits).
- *Certificate*: Anyone can issue a certificate. The same principles apply as for the diploma (see above).
- *APEL (Accreditation of Prior Experiential Learning)*: This acknowledges that traditional classroom-based learning is not the only way of gaining knowledge normally associated with textbooks and classroom teaching. Experiential learning is that which we learn from experience – not simply doing the same thing again and again, but while undertaking something in clinical practice. This could involve searching the literature, writing procedures or publishing findings. If such experiential learning can be matched to a specific module of study at a university, then students may be able to provide the evidence that they have achieved the module outcomes by an alternative route.
- *APL (Accreditation of Prior Learning)*: This is similar to APEL, but is focused on another educational institution being the source of learning. Thus someone may have undertaken a module of study on research methods while on a health studies degree. When undertaking a post-registration specialist nursing degree, the person may put in a claim that they have already met the outcomes of the specialist nursing research methods module.
- *APA (Accreditation of Prior Achievement)*: This is a general term that is usually used to cover both APEL and APL, as most claims involve both APEL and APL.
- *CAT (Credit Accumulation and Transfer) points*: This covers the same ideas as in APEL, APL and APA, but it specifically means the transfer

of a module of learning from one course or university to the course you are undertaking. Each course and university has individual regulations as to how, if at all, they allow this. Most courses will allow 20–25% of level 4 credits to be transferred in from other universities. However, at level 6 this is reduced to 15%, if it is allowed at all.

- *Advanced standing*: The normal structure for a degree is to start at year one on level 4 and work through to the end of year three. Advanced standing is the acceptance of students onto year two or year three of the degree, based upon previous APEL and/or APA. The most common example of this for nurses can be found in post-registration degrees. Most pre-registration education gives the nurse a Diploma in Higher Education (Nursing) with their professional registration. Most universities that run pre-registration nursing courses at diploma level will also have a post-registration degree that allows advanced standing from pre-registration Diplomas in Higher Education (Nursing). Thus nurses may undertake pre-registration education in one part of the country and then move to another part of the country. In their new location, they enrol on a degree course that allows them to transfer in their Diploma in Higher Education (Nursing) (240 credits) via advanced standing and then complete the equivalent of the third year of the degree.

CAT and APL are complicated yet extremely valuable structures, which many nurses can utilise. If you feel that you have credits or experience that could form part of your further studies, then seek out someone at your local university who understands the course regulations regarding APA. This may take a bit of detective work on your part, but it will be well worth the effort.

What is involved in reflective practice?

Claire Agnew

Learning is not achieved solely by having an experience or attending a study day. Learning is a result of thought and consideration – reflection about what the experience actually meant to you. The ability to reflect effectively is fundamental to the development of nursing (Andrews, 1996). Reflection is also an important part of reviewing your strengths and weaknesses and identifying areas that need developing. It means thinking about an event, analysing what occurred, what your thoughts and feelings were about the event, and identifying what you did well and what you could learn from it. Reflection can take place in a variety of ways: a reflective journal, portfolio development, structured sessions, or the use of a framework (Hulatt, 1995).

Situations that you should reflect upon include:

- Something you enjoyed or went well.
- Something you found difficult to deal with.
- A situation where things went wrong.
- A crisis or emergency.
- Something you do every day.
- Something you rarely do.

(Jarvis, 1992; Haddock and Bassett, 1997; Johns, 2000)

How to reflect

How you choose to reflect upon your practice and experiences is a personal decision, although it is recommended that you choose a model that will guide you through the stages of reflective learning. Sharing your reflections with someone you feel comfortable with may provide another way of looking at the situation. Gibbs' reflective cycle (1988; *Figure 5.3*) provides a simple approach to reflection. *Figure 5.4* shows a framework that you may find useful. It is important to see reflection in practice as an important way of developing your nursing practice and not just an academic exercise.

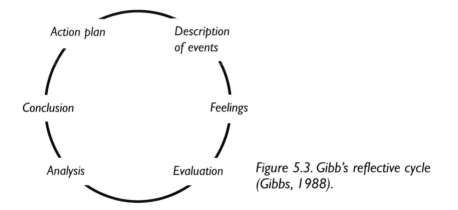

Figure 5.3. Gibb's reflective cycle (Gibbs, 1988).

Description (what happened?)
Feelings (What were you thinking and feeling?) and evaluation (What was good and bad about the experience?)
Analysis (What sense can you make of the situation?)
Conclusion (What else could you have done?)
Action plan and learning outcome
Signature

Figure 5.4. Framework for reflection using the reflective cycle.

How do I prepare for an interview?
Claire Agnew

Creating the right impression at interview takes preparation. For some jobs you may be the only applicant. Other jobs may have 10 or 20 applicants for one position. No job will be yours automatically. You need to find ways of getting the edge over other applicants, and that means preparation and presentation.

Getting an interview is reliant on your application form; it needs to be concise and comprehensive. When I shortlist candidates for interview, I look for good clear presentation. Obvious presentation points are very important, yet often missed:

- Do not write your application form in blue ink when they ask for black.
- Ensure that your handwriting is legible.
- Fill in all the sections.

I also expect to see the supporting statement box filled with personal qualities:

- What you have done outside work that could have a positive effect on your practice.
- Insight into the role you are applying for, and not just 'I want to work on a cardiac ward to increase my skills in dealing with cardiac arrests'.
- I am looking for someone who is going to be motivated, demonstrate commitment and fit into the team.

Pointers for interviews

When you get an interview, go on an informal visit where appropriate, or if it is a promotion within your existing area, arrange to see the senior nurse, training and development team or the management team. This will give you the opportunity to find out others' expectations of the role that you are applying for and aid your preparation; it will also help you demonstrate your interest and commitment. The Royal College of Nursing and the *Nursing Times* websites offer very practical advice on interview preparation and preparing your CV or application form. See the boxes for some pointers for interviews and for lists of questions you may be asked at interview.

If you are unsuccessful, try not to be too disappointed. The more sought after or senior the job, the greater will be the interest and competition. Try to learn from the experience, both in terms of your character and also from how you could improve next time. Most interviewers will give you the opportunity to receive feedback; if this is not offered to you, then ask. Try to treat it positively and make sure that you are willing to listen, learn and develop.

Pointers for interviews

- Arrive in good time: this will allow you to collect your thoughts
- Research the role you are applying for
- Dress smartly – you are a professional
- Read the job description thoroughly and think through what the role involves
- Think of some possible scenarios that you may be asked; where possible, answer them with previous experiences that you have learnt from
- Think of some questions to ask the panel
- Take your professional profile and offer it to the panel to look at

---

Questions you may be asked at interview

- Why do you want this job?
- How do you deal with stress?
- What is important to you as a nurse?
- What do you understand by the term clinical supervision?
- What do you understand by the term clinical governance?
- What do you understand by (insert any current Government initiative or publication)?
- What qualities do you possess that you can bring to this role?
- Who or what has most inspired you?
- Tell me about a recent article you have read that has influenced your practice.

What is the role of the mentor?

Paul Pleasance and Deborah Dowsett

There is now a much greater emphasis on the support of students undertaking placements in the clinical setting than used to be the case (Department of Health, 2000a, 2000b; English National Board for Nursing, Midwifery and Health Visiting, 2001). Due to the nature of rapid change taking place in healthcare and nursing in general, the role of the registered nurse when supporting student nurses in the practice setting has been recently reviewed and to give it greater clarity and direction. The NMC (2006/2008) has been instrumental in providing clear standards for mentors to support the leaning and assessment of student nurses in the practice setting which have replaced previously existing standards (NMC, 2008).

In the clinical setting a variety of new roles has developed, all of which have become allied to support the education of the student nurse or more junior nurse undertaking additional post-registration professional development and further education courses. These roles include practice (or clinical) experience coordinators, sign off mentors, lecturer practitioners, clinical educators, training leads, practice educators and practice teachers In some areas the contribution of senior students to supporting more junior students has also been officially recognised through the use of 'buddying systems'.

However, there is little doubt that the most important people in the everyday practice-based life of nursing students are still the staff nurses. They are there, all the time, working as the registered nurse in the clinical setting and fulfilling the role to which the student aspires. It is staff nurses who are likely to be allocated the task of 'looking after' the student. So- how do you do it? What skills do you need? And how can those skills be developed?

First, it may be helpful to clear up a few misconceptions and give some working definitions of the different types of assessors that you may come across within the clinical area.

Mentors

Generally speaking, nursing students can and will be supervised by a whole range of professionals during the course of their studies, including nurses, midwives, social workers, teachers, play therapists, operating department practitioners and doctors. All of these people, provided that they understand the nature, type and content of the nursing curriculum, can make an important contribution to the learning experience of the student. While those professionals who are not first-level registered nurses can also contribute to the assessment of students (by providing feedback, for example), the formal assessment of achievement of nursing competence and proficiency must be completed by a first-level registered nurse who has undergone further preparation and training to fulfil the role of mentor and so will function as the formal assessor. This is the person whom the NMC (2008) now refers to as a 'mentor'.

An NMC mentor is a registrant who, following successful completion of an NMC approved mentor preparation programme, has achieved the knowledge, skills and competence required.

A mentor is a mandatory requirement for pre-registration nursing students. In case there is any doubt left in your mind, as you look back at your own nurse education programme, remember that all students are responsible for their own actions and inactions, but cannot be professionally accountable for those actions until they are registered. This means that the person who is supervising the student effectively carries that burden. It would be useful therefore to distinguish in your mind the difference between direct supervision and indirect supervision. Indirect supervision reflects the fact that once the supervisor (and the student) are both confident in the ability of the student to carry out specific duties, the student can go and do them without having somebody looking over her/his shoulder (but the supervisor is still accountable for the student's actions). If the student and/or supervisor are not confident about the required activity, then it is essential that the student is directly supervised until both parties are happy about it.

There are other situations, e.g. the checking or administration of drugs (so long as this is permissible under local policy), when the student should only ever be allowed to work under direct supervision – in other words, even if the student becomes quite skilled at it, she/he cannot do it alone until fully registered.

Sign off mentors

The sign off mentor is required in pre-registration nursing for students who are on final placements, or for post-registration students who are on approved specialist practice programmes leading to a registrable or recordable award with the NMC (2008).

Before you become a sign off mentor you have to demonstrate that you have met the sign off mentor criteria set by the NMC (2008) in full, including having been supervised on at least three occasions for signing off proficiency (at the end of a final placement) by an existing sign off mentor before being annotated as such on the local mentor register.

Practice teachers

An NMC practice teacher is a registered nurse who has previously fulfilled the NMC requirements to become a mentor and who has taken further preparation to achieve the knowledge and skills along with the competence required to meet the NMC defined outcomes for a practice teacher. The NMC requires all students working towards registration as a Specialist Community Public Health Nurse (SCPHN) to have a named practice teacher.

Preparation of mentors

Until August 2001, there was no standard or universal pattern for the preparation of supervisors and assessors of pre-registration nursing students. There was a variety of courses, ranging from the ENB 998 Teaching and Assessing in Clinical Practice through to individual study days. Since 1 September 2001, all of that officially ceased with the introduction of the new Preparation of Mentors programme, which replaced the ENB 997/998 and, for community staff, the Community Practice Teacher course. Since then mentor preparation courses have been given much more definition and clarity by the NMC (2004, 2008). A register of mentors who have undergone a further preparation course is held by the local placement provider (subject to regular updating and continued professional development/registration) to enable students to be placed with appropriately trained mentors. Nurses who are not on the register of mentors and assessors now have to undertake the new courses before they can be the official named mentor for nursing students. Obviously, you will need to check out local information about the course in your area, but some of the standard criteria for a mentor to take on the role include:

- Being registered in the same part or sub-part of the register as the student they are to assess.
- Being registered in the same part or sub-part of the register as the student they are to assess and the same field of practice.
- Having developed their own knowledge skills and competence beyond registration, i.e. having been registered for at least a year.
- Having successfully completed an NMC approved mentor preparation programme.
- Being able to make judgements about competence and proficiency of NMC students and be accountable for their decisions (NMC, 2008).

While widely welcomed, these changes have created some new challenges for all the stakeholders in the nursing education process. The most significant challenge is perhaps that, with the best will in the world, in many areas the new preparation of mentors courses simply cannot, in the short-term, prepare enough new mentors to meet the demand. This has led to including the development of distance/open learning versions of the course. Furthermore, the valued contribution that continues to be made by professional nurses (and others) who are not recognised mentors has been acknowledged by the introduction of concepts such as team mentoring and associate or secondary mentors. These are professionals who have undergone some basic preparation for the role and are able to supervise nursing students with confidence, and who contribute to the assessment process by providing feedback to both the student and to the named mentor, but it is the named mentor who has undergone formal preparation who should then complete the formal part of the assessment.

Arguably this section might be seen as underpinning the preparation that associate or secondary mentors might receive, but hopefully it will provide some back-up and revision for people who are doing, or have done, the full mentor preparation programme.

Mentoring a student

We know that the mentor is a person who facilitates learning and supervises and assesses students while they are undergoing practice experience. But what does this mean in real terms? Lloyd Jones et al (2001) add 'general support' and 'acting as a role model' to the list, and also make the point that the word mentor is probably a misnomer, since the relationship between mentor and student is inevitably too short-lived to be really meaningful (being limited by the duration of the placement). Neary et al (1994) describe a good mentor as someone who possesses appropriate professional attributes, knowledge and good communication skills, and has the motivation to teach and support students. There is perhaps a distinction between informal and formal mentoring. Undoubtedly the statutory body is talking about the latter, but it would be inappropriate not to acknowledge, in our professional practice, the importance of the former, i.e. informal mentoring. If we accept this, and see mentoring as a positive endeavour we might then add other dimensions to the role – such as knowledgeable friend, helper, advocate, challenger (Earnshaw, 1995; Cahill, 1996), coach, counsellor and guide (Morton-Cooper and Palmer, 1993) and perhaps even confidante (Glen and Parker, 2003).

Creating a relationship

It may be considered obvious that the quality of the relationship between the student and the mentor is vital if mentorship is to be successful. However,

Jarvis and Gibson (1997) suggest that the relationship does not have to be of a certain type in order for this to take place – arguably the relationship might be as informal or formal as the types of mentoring that take place. They conclude that:

Mentorship is about exercising this characteristic [openness] in genuine dialogue, so that ultimately both [the mentor and the student] develop and feel needed through the relationship.

One of the most important aspects of building the relationship and making mentorship work is regular contact (Lloyd Jones et al, 2001) so that the two parties can start to feel comfortable and confident about each other. The most obvious way is to try to ensure that you work together as frequently as possible, especially if the student is able to work alongside you while you are involved in giving care. This approach has three benefits:

- It allows the student to learn by observing first hand.
- It demonstrates to the student that you have sufficient confidence in your own skills and are happy to have those skills scrutinised.
- It can begin to demonstrate that you trust and respect the student as a colleague.

Opportunities to work together are made easier by the fact that it is now usual for the student to experience care across the full 24-hour, seven day a week timespan from very early in their course. So, with appropriate negotiation, it should be possible to go some way towards having matching duty schedules. This also helps to fulfil the statutory obligation that the mentor is required to:

...use knowledge of the student's stage of learning to select appropriate opportunities to meet individual needs.

(NMC, 2008: 20)

On the other hand, the assessment focus and the need to 'get the signature in the box' (and the implicit 'power' dynamics that this imposes) can distort the relationship and make it hard for the student to be honest, open and to admit to shortfalls in knowledge. Care is clearly needed to keep a balance between the various components of the role and to ensure that the relationship is a healthy one.

In a report of her research into effective mentoring, Spouse (1996) suggested ways in which the relationship between the mentor and student can be optimised. These included such basic things as the mentor initiating social interactions, which, as well as promoting trust, show a sense of warmth – in other words, having a chat and demonstrating a personal interest in the student while, at the same time, being able and willing to share her/his own personal feelings and experiences and thus being seen as a real person in the student's eyes. Spouse (1996) also found that student stress was inversely proportional to the degree of student familiarity and friendliness demonstrated by the mentor.

Gray and Smith (2000) summarised this neatly when they concluded that having a good mentor usually coincides with having a good placement. Rather more anecdotally, it is worth noting that I regularly have cause to ask students about their practical experiences and specifically about what they believe constitutes a good practice placement; the answers consistently come back along the following lines:

- 'They actually knew that I existed and were expecting me.'
- 'My mentor made me feel welcome and took an interest in me.'
- 'They seemed to like having students and wanted to teach me.'
- 'They were always willing to ask me questions, and help me find out the answers if I didn't know.'
- 'They didn't mind me asking questions or feel threatened by me asking them.'
- 'They really know their stuff on that ward.'
- 'They didn't just leave the students to fend for themselves.'
- 'Even when they were busy, they didn't make me feel like a nuisance.'

Perhaps equally significant in these days of staff shortages and difficulties in filling vacancies, such discussions with students often end with:

- 'I'd love to go back there to work as a staff nurse.'

Relationships between students and mentors can be important for all sorts of reasons.

In conclusion of this section, the suggestions arising from the research by Gray and Smith (2000) into the qualities of a good mentor (as perceived by student nurses) make a helpful checklist:

- Enthusiastic.
- Friendly.
- Approachable.
- Patient and understanding.
- Good sense of humour.
- Good role model.

- Professional and organised.
- Caring and self-confident.
- Good communicator.
- Knowledgeable about the student's course.
- Has realistic expectations of (plus confidence and trust in) the student's abilities.
- Provides regular feedback.
- Involves the student in activities.
- Spends time with the student.
- Shows a genuine interest in the student.
- Is willing and able gradually to reduce the level of direct supervision.

No-one said that being a mentor was going to be easy.

Liaising with the university

It now seems to be more widely accepted that nursing education is a shared activity between the university and the practice environment; it is not just the case that the university's students have to spend 50% of their course in practice.

Perhaps more importantly, it is no longer perceived that the university 'does the theory side' and the wards 'do the practice side'. The shared ownership for the education and training of nurses has resulted in an increase in teamwork between the two sides, which itself is leading to an enhanced understanding of each other's respective needs. This is a state of affairs that we all want to encourage. However, it may be confusing to know who to contact at the university and when. Safe bets it will be either the module leader or the programme leader. If the names and telephone numbers are not recorded on the front of the assessment document or module guide that the student should have presented to you, then ask the student to record it – before there is a need to do so. The bottom line is that it does not really matter who you contact at the university if you have concerns about a student (or if you want to say how wonderful he/she is), but be prepared to be referred on to the right person. Please do not let that put you off. It really is important that communication between the university and yourself in the clinical setting supporting students, continues.

It is also important to remember that there is a range of people who might be able to deal with any queries you may have in connection with students and their course. People such as practice experience coordinators, lecturer/practitioners and allocations officers can be useful contacts. It is also not uncommon for university departments of nursing to identify specific lecturers to link with individual directorates or units. If you are not sure who your 'link lecturer' is, again it would be worth finding out and then making use of her or him.

Giving feedback

Formal assessment of students will be examined at a later stage in this chapter. Formative assessment is usually defined as the provision of feedback on a student's progress, which is not used to make specific judgements about the student passing or failing. A typical example of a formative assessment might be:

> *When you carried out that bedbath on Mr X I noticed you paid particular attention to maintaining his dignity and privacy. But when we do it tomorrow, perhaps we can focus on the importance of observing and recording the state of his skin at the same time.*

It is ironic that, generally speaking, we find it easier to give praise than to criticise, and yet students often report that they do not get any feedback except about their failings – and then often too late for them to be able to do anything about it to put things right. Two golden rules about giving feedback might be seen to emerge from this last statement:

- Do not hesitate to provide positive feedback and praise on a student's performance, i.e. do not rely on the maxim, 'No news is good news'.
- If things are not going well, then make sure the student knows about it as early as possible.

The objective here is to ensure that the student has as much time as possible to put matters right and, hopefully, avoid failing an assessment. Incidentally, you might consider it good practice to let the module leader at the university know at the same time so that she or he can support the student (and you) early on as well.

Students want and need feedback on both their strengths and weaknesses. They cannot engage in effective reflection and thereby refocus their learning if they do not know how well they are doing. So long as the relationship is built on mutual trust and respect (as discussed earlier), students value constructive criticism about their knowledge, skills and attitudes. The proviso is that any such feedback should be discreet and take place away from the patient (Spouse, 1996) and other members of staff.

Having made this last point, it is only fair to point out that as the mentor of the student, you will receive feedback from other members of the team (with whom the student may have worked while you were not there).

It will take skill and courage to talk to the student about issues and concerns that are 'secondhand' while ensuring that the student is convinced of the professional value of other supervisors reporting their opinions to you. Consideration could be given to whether the advantages of negotiating a 'ward' philosophy whereby, wherever practical, only the named mentor should provide detailed feedback to the student outweigh the disadvantages. However it is acknowledged that, sometimes, feedback cannot wait and has to be given immediately.

What is involved in teaching a student?

Paul Pleasance and Deborah Dowsett

One of the aspects of the role of mentor most valued by the student is the teaching component, and this is a theme that recurs throughout the research literature concerning mentorship of student nurses (e.g. Spouse, 1996; Andrews and Chilton, 2000; Gray and Smith, 2000). Students realise that there is much more to teaching than being taken away from the ward environment, perhaps to an empty side ward or day room, and being sat down to receive a lecture from one of the ward team. That is not to say that there is not a place for this on occasions: there undoubtedly is, and students enjoy it. But it is not the most important part of teaching, even though some of the principles outlined in subsequent sections might apply equally well to formal and informal teaching opportunities.

Setting learning outcomes

In the world of education the relative merits of 'objectives' versus 'outcomes' have been debated for many years. My personal feeling is that using the term 'outcomes' is probably more helpful because it encourages you to focus on what the student should learn (i.e. student-centred) rather than what the teacher should teach (teacher-centred) or what the student should be able to do (behavioural objectives).

But that is all just semantics. What is important is that consideration should be given to identifying the learning needs of the student and the learning opportunities provided by the practice placement environment.

The first question might be, 'What is the student here for?' The simplest answer would be to learn how to 'do' nursing – the practice side of it. After all (you might argue), the university is there to provide the theory part. But that would undervalue your expertise as a staff nurse/mentor. You do not just know about the practical side. You are the expert with the theoretical underpinnings.

So, have the confidence to see yourself as an expert (that is not the same as suggesting that you know everything): teaching a student is about being able to share that expertise – the theory and the practice. It is a reasonable expectation that students should be able to specify what they want and/or need to learn while allocated to your area (if not, send them away to come back the next day, having identified some of their intentions). The university will have provided some guidance to the students regarding what they might expect to get out of the experience. Conversely, it is also a reasonable expectation that you will be able to identify the general and unique learning opportunities that your practice environment can provide (if not, sit down with your colleagues and do the exercise – then include your conclusions in the induction pack that you provide for all students on their first day on the ward (you do have one, don't you?). Once you have identified the learning needs of the student, and the learning opportunities of the placement, identifying learning outcomes is a marriage between the two. Of course, you will need to take into account a range of other issues to set the context of this exercise, for example:

- How long is the student to be placed with you?
- What stage of the course is the student at?
- What patients are you looking after at the moment?
- Are you planning an individual teaching session, or a day of supervised practice, or the whole allocation?
- What assessment objectives have been set that the student will have to meet?

The main value of identifying anticipated learning outcomes is that it ensures that all the players in the game – the student, you and the other members of the caring team – know and understand the purpose of the allocation. Learning outcomes can also be used to show everybody what they can contribute to the student's learning. In summary:

- Learning outcomes should reflect the match between what the student wants and/or needs to know, and what learning opportunities are presented by the practice experience.

The next stage is to give some thought to how to ensure that the student achieves the agreed learning outcomes.

The learning environment

Most of our students do want to learn. Although the way they present themselves and voice their desires may be different from what we expect, the majority are still highly vocationally oriented and want to learn all the things necessary for them to become good professional nurses. This goes a long way towards ensuring solid, intrinsic motivation to learn, as opposed to the extrinsic types of motivation borne only out of such things as obligation, compulsion and fear of failure.

The classic work of Maslow (1943) would have us believe that, before effective new learning can take place, all other more basic needs should be dealt with. Despite its age, Maslow's hierarchy of needs still provides a useful template for assessing the learning environment and reminding the teacher of the considerations necessary to create a setting that will ensure that optimal learning can occur. As further clues, a review of the literature, coupled with a discussion with students, provides the following list of the characteristics of a positive learning environment. Any person who wants to teach in a practice setting will be challenged by the following list.

- A welcoming atmosphere.
- The provision of high quality, evidence-based care.
- Repeated opportunity to practise skills under supervision.
- A willingness to ask and answer questions.
- A willingness to repeat explanations – once is rarely enough.
- Skilled, competent and confident practitioners who act as role models.
- Clear and effective links with the educational institution.
- Recognition by staff of student learning needs.
- Effective team leadership and good staff relations.
- Time dedicated to teaching – including the use of 'quiet time'.

It is no coincidence that there is much common ground between the above list and the characteristics of good mentors and good placements discussed earlier. However, one of the most significant obstacles to professional learning reported by students is that they are sometimes not sure about what they need to know. If students do not know what they need to know, it is unlikely that they will be able to identify and utilise learning opportunities effectively. It sometimes happens, then, that those students end up repeating the same activities over and over again, and fail to move on to develop other skills and knowledge.

Learning resources

In one sense, the learning environment is, or should be, an important learning resource. Knowles (1980) summarises it as follows:

> The psychological climate should be one which causes adults to feel accepted, respected and supported; in which there exists a spirit of mutuality between teachers and students as joint enquirers; in which there is freedom of expression without fear of punishment or ridicule.

There are basically three learning resources open to the student undertaking a practice experience in your area:

- You (as the student's mentor).
- Other members of the interprofessional caring team.

- The environment of practice itself – specifically, the patients who are there to be cared for.

This last point might create some potential ethical dilemmas since it infers that patients are being used for professional purposes, which of course they are. The fact that students are supervised in their practice effectively eliminates many of the ethical concerns, but theoretically patients can decline to have students of any kind contribute to their care delivery.

It is the role of the mentor to plan and coordinate the student's experience to ensure the best opportunities to capitalise upon what those three learning resources can offer; and if there appear to be gaps in the range of opportunities that exist, then the mentor can often create and utilise alternatives. This might mean, for example, organising activities so that the student can:

- Spend some or all of a shift in a different area.
- Work with specific people with specific expertise.
- Observe techniques or procedures.
- Escort a patient.
- Follow a patient journey.
- Follow up some new practice experience with some theory input.
- Go to the library to obtain evidence to support a practice intervention.

There is another resource that students can learn from – which nurses tend to shun in their search for professional respectability – and that is knowledge derived from the history and culture of nursing. Practitioners need not be afraid of this kind of knowledge, especially when that culture embraces the concept of evidence. These are things that students cannot gain from a classroom or a book, but they are things that the professional practice-based mentor is uniquely placed to help the student to learn.

Approaches to teaching

It is beyond the scope of this chapter to try to deliver a teacher training programme that would attempt to teach mentors how to teach their students. What can be achieved is probably to provide some pointers that might form a basis for reflection, out of which the mentor may start to develop a personal philosophy of how to tackle student teaching – especially within the context of some of the earlier sections under the heading of 'Teaching a student'. For instance, it has become popular in the past 20 years or so for educationalists to debate the relative merits of pedagogy (which traditionally was used to describe the art and science of teaching, but now tends to be reserved for the teaching of children) and androgogy, which is usually reserved to describe the art and science of teaching adults.

Knowles (1973) was one of the first to describe such a theory and concluded that adults learn best when:

- The learning is self-directed.
- The learning is related to their past experience.
- Whatever is to be learned is relevant to their everyday life.
- The learning material is of a problem-solving nature.

Despite the number of years ago that these findings were first recorded, and the subsequent arguments that the differences between adult and children learning are not as clearly polarised as they might suggest, there is undoubtedly much that can and should be learned from these points.

In an ideal world, whenever we are faced with a new student, we should undertake some kind of learning styles inventory; this would enable us to make an assessment of how we should set out to teach (or facilitate the learning of) that individual student. In reality that is probably not practical, but the only thing about which there is certainty is that the student is an adult (rather than a child).

An observation may be that there might be something about nursing and nurses (and, in fairness, probably about departments of nursing in universities) that causes us to tend to feel more comfortable slightly further along the continuum towards pedagogy than might be the case of other professional student groups. So do not be afraid to go down that route if it seems appropriate. The important thing is to get to know the student, so that you both feel comfortable enough within the relationship to allow flexibility in the way that things are taught – and learned.

A final point under the heading of 'approach to teaching'. Whatever approach you decide is appropriate, the emphasis needs to be upon 'learning'. You can teach and facilitate all day, but if the student is not learning, it is a complete waste of time.

What is involved in assessing a student?
Paul Pleasance and Deborah Dowsett

The good part about assessing students is that it acknowledges their achievements and shows how they have progressed towards the goal of registration. The bad part is that students sometimes fail. We will look at that a little later.

Formative assessment

This was defined earlier as the provision of feedback on a student's progress, which is not used to make specific judgements about the student passing or failing.

Summative assessment

Conversely, this is the judgment that students either pass or fail, and which is therefore used to form the basis of whether or not they can progress on their course and, ultimately, qualify as a nurse.

Characteristics of assessment

Each university department of nursing is required to formulate, in collaboration with colleagues from the service, assessment tools for both the theory and practice components of the course. There is a shared commitment to ensuring that all assessments are:

- *Valid*: They do assess what they are supposed to assess.
- *Reliable*: The outcomes of assessment are consistent, irrespective of when the assessment takes place and who completes it.
- *Discriminating*: A 'good' student will pass and a 'bad' student will fail.
- *Practical*: The conduct of the assessment is reasonable in terms of what it demands of the assessor by way of resources, such as time and money. It is not uncommon now for practice-based staff to be involved in the theory-based assessment of students, but it is much more likely that you will be involved in assessing the practice competence of your students.

Part of your preparation to undertake the role of mentor, and part of your annual updating, should include developing an understanding of the nature, kind, content and use of the assessment documents used by the university in your area. If there is any doubt in your mind about what specifically is required of you, then please contact a member of the university staff (see earlier section on liaising with the university) or other relevant person for guidance – before you need it. Saying to the student, 'What am I supposed to do with this?' as she/he hands you the assessment book does not inspire the kind of confidence that is required as a basis for a healthy mentor/student relationship.

What is assessed?

Whichever university you are working with, you will find certain things in common. For example, all assessment documents will monitor and record the student's ongoing achievement in:

- Practical skills.
- Intellectual skills.
- Interpersonal skills, including:
    - ability to work within a team
    - ability to relate to patients and their families.
- Integration of theory and practice.
- Professionalism/professional conduct.

Pitfalls in assessment

The onus is on the mentor to try to ensure that the assessment is undertaken as fairly and objectively as possible. One of the advantages of concepts such as team mentoring is that it helps to share the load of the responsibility a little: because no single mentor will be able to work with the student all the time that she/he is on duty, the wise mentor will seek and receive feedback from other members of the team, perhaps associate or secondary mentors (see earlier), on how the student has performed in relation to the above areas of achievement. In the end, however, it is the mentor who has the final say as to whether or not the student has achieved the standard of performance required.

It may therefore be worth considering briefly some of the pitfalls in assessment that the mentor will need to avoid:

- *First impressions*: Sometimes the first impression formed of an individual can distort later perceptions, e.g. if the student is late on the first day, however genuine the reason, this can cause people to make wrong assumptions about other aspects of performance.
- *Halo effect*: This is where one feature or characteristic exhibited by the student (good or bad) influences or inhibits later observations, e.g.

great sporting prowess, physical characteristics.

- *Stereotyping*: This is where we subconsciously classify new experiences of persons using assumptions 'learned' in the past. Most of us have to make conscious efforts not to make generalised and inappropriate assumptions about groups of people. As an example, reflect for a minute on how the general public tends to characterise nurses.
- *Recency effect*: In this situation, our overall view of a person is coloured by our most recent interactions with them. Thus, if a nurse performs badly today, we can be tempted to overlook the fact that she/ he performed perfectly adequately on every preceding day, and that there may be a reason for today's performance.
- *Interpersonal attraction*: We are not talking lust here; just that if someone appeals to you, whether physically or emotionally, or if they seem to like you, then that fact can potentially influence your objectivity and make you view other aspects of their work more favourably (of course, the opposite to attraction can be equally powerful).
- *Self-fulfilling prophecy*: Eventually, it seems, people tend to behave how others expect them to. This is commonly seen in children, but many of us have experienced it in adult life. We do well if we are expected to do well; a student turns out to be useless if that is the expectation given to you (and them) by their previous assessor.

Purposes of assessment

Nobody would argue with the mentor that assessment of students is an onerous responsibility, which is in no way reduced when consideration is given to the reasons why assessment is carried out in the first place:

- To provide the student with feedback on progress.
- To motivate the student to achieve outcomes.
- To indicate the effectiveness of instruction.
- To indicate the effectiveness of the curriculum.

These reasons are usually fairly easy to cope with and are unlikely to cause too much stress. However, it would be a dereliction of duty not to mention the observation that, whenever a student fails to achieve, it is always necessary for the 'teacher' (whether university-based or practice-based) to investigate the cause and to ensure that the performance is not in some way a reflection of the quality of support that the student is receiving.

What happens if a student is failing?

The next two reasons for assessment which potentially cause some degree of anxiety because so much depends on them are:

- To indicate to the statutory body the suitability of the student to be licensed.
- To safeguard the standards of nursing care and health and wellbeing of the public by maintaining a satisfactory level of fitness to practice in future practitioners.

These are not responsibilities that anyone could take lightly. It does, however, beg the question: what happens if the student fails? Perhaps the first point to note is that it is a difficult decision to fail a student, and it can be uncomfortable and unpleasant. We all accept that there are times when it is the only option, but that does not make it any easier.

Remember that assessment is a shared activity between you and the university (and the student). So, an important point is not to feel you are on your own. Do not even just keep it among your colleagues in the placement area, make sure you discuss your concerns with appropriate staff from the university as soon as you have doubts that your student will succeed for whatever reason. This then leads to the other golden rule of assessment, namely that a failed assessment should not come as a surprise to anybody – not the student, not the other members of the ward team, and not the university.

As part of the ongoing mentoring process, it is essential that a failure to make satisfactory progress is highlighted as early as possible, so that you and the student can sit down together to draw up an action plan (in conjunction with a member of the module team from the university) designed to help students to overcome their weaknesses and, ultimately, to achieve the objectives, i.e. to help students to pass.

If and when, having tried everything in your power, you do have to fail your student, it may strike you that when your last 25 students all passed satisfactorily, you never heard a word from the university. Now you have failed someone, people are suddenly contacting you. Do not be alarmed or surprised by this. It does not imply any criticism of you or your decision, and it certainly should not be interpreted as pressure being brought to bear upon you to pass this student (or future students). If I were the module leader, or the programme leader, the main reason why I would contact you would be to ensure that I had a full and complete picture of all the circumstances to present to the Assessment Board so that I could support your recommendation with confidence and authority.

It may make you feel a little better to learn that it is unlikely to be the end of the line for the student. There will be options for retrieval, although it has to be acknowledged that even final attempts are sometimes failed.

Discussing actions to take when failing a student may seem like a very negative note upon which to conclude a consideration of the ways in which practice staff can support nursing students. Thankfully, it is very much the exception rather than the rule, and the majority of students do make the grade, so long as they are given clear guidance of what is expected of them. On a positive note, general feedback within my area of work suggests that mentors feel empowered in their role and enthused by the opportunity which they have to make a vital contribution to the education and training of nurses. Mentors, sign off mentors and practice teachers play a major role in enhancing student learning at whatever level. They act as role models, perform socialisation roles, and act as assessors to provide quality learning and teaching in the clinical environment. This they see as an investment in their own future and a chance to positively influence the caring and professional ability not only of their students but for the profession as a whole.

What are my roles and responsibilities regarding the Mental Health Act?

Paul Rigby

While it is understandable to assume that roles and responsibilities relating to the Mental Health Act will concern only mental health and learning disability nurses, there are situations where nurses outside these specialties will have contact with patients subject to such legislation.

The Mental Health Act (1983/2007) provides a legislative framework that enables people with a mental disorder to receive care and treatment. The vast majority of people accessing mental healthcare in inpatient settings do so on an informal basis; however, there are some who, for a variety of reasons, require legal compulsion to ensure that care and treatment are received. It is important to remember that the power to give treatment that the Act provides applies only to treatment for a mental disorder. The power to treat may be applied to a physical treatment if it is in some way related to the mental disorder, although this is not common practice and is a complex legal area.

Nurses will have contact with people who are suffering from a mental disorder such as a severe depressive illness, who will sometimes present for treatment in an accident and emergency department following an episode of self-harm. If they are willing to give their consent to treatment this is usually provided before they are referred to a specialist mental health practitioner.

If this consent is withheld or withdrawn, it is important to remember that treatment can still be provided under common law provided that treatment is necessary to save life, prevent suffering or prevent deterioration in the patient's condition (Mental Health Act, 1983, 2007). This is a complex area of practice and requires good communication, effective teamwork and strong leadership.

People who are detained under the Mental Health Act will require treatment in non-mental health inpatient settings, such as a medical or surgical ward, and in such circumstances specialist nurses will provide continuous support. The responsibilities for the nurse in such circumstances revolve around the provision of care and treatment for the physical condition only. However, the principles of effective networking with other care providers; good teamwork, including the setting of clear boundaries in relation to roles and responsibilities; and good communication, are essential if effective holistic care is to be provided.

How do I refer patients to the community services?
Tracey Kemmett and John Fowler

General principles when referring or discharging patients

Good communication and early planning is the key to all referrals and discharges. When you are new to an area the paperwork and general systems can be a little confusing and not every area has a clear step-by-step process identified. However, each service will have a specific referral form that will need to be completed. Find out where these forms are located, what information is required and where they need to be sent once they are completed. Ensure that the referral is recorded in the patient's documentation, including the date, whom the referral has been sent to, and your signature and designation.

When should I refer patients to the community services?

This depends on the patient's health needs. If the patient has relatively simple requirements, such as suture removal, the referral can be carried out the day before discharge during the normal working week (Monday to Friday). If the patient is being discharged at a weekend or beginning of a bank holiday period, the service may be limited, so ensure that the referral is carried out with at least one working day's notice. If in doubt, contact those who will be providing the care and ask for advice. Make sure you find out all you can regarding any specific points that are relevant to your particular clinical speciality and 'peculiar' to your local area. Some staff for instance like the paperwork completed and a telephone conversation (there is only so much information you can convey in writing). So make sure you pick the brains of the more experienced staff in your area.

If the patient's needs are complex or particularly specialised, early referral to the community services is essential. Continuing healthcare is where health needs are beyond that which is normally expected, e.g. visits from a district nurse three times a week.

The assessment, which is usually performed by a registered nurse, will start the process for obtaining specialist equipment or particular care such as 24-hour home nursing. This documentation should ask key questions that identify health needs or requirements for assessment by the multidisciplinary team.

More complex care may require input from social services as well as the health services. Contacting all who need to be involved as early as possible will reduce the chance of finding something that has not been addressed on the day of discharge, which could result in a delay in the patient's discharge.

Why refer patients to the community services?

An admission to hospital may identify or create the need for additional care support once the patient returns home. An assessment carried out on a patient's admission to hospital may reveal that patients are not coping in their current home environment, or that the effects of operative intervention or illness will affect their ability to achieve a reasonable quality of life safely.

- So, what would that patient need?
- Imagine how the patient would cope if you were to send them home the next day.
- Assessing the full picture is vital; think about the everyday activities that the patient may need assistance with and who could provide this.

Appropriate referral depends on accurate needs assessment of the patient and knowledge of the systems and services available locally. If sutures need removing, a practice nurse can do this, or if the patient is unable to get to the GP, then a visit from a district nurse will need to be arranged. If the patient has complex needs that require frequent nursing intervention, the district nurse may wish to visit and assess the patient before discharge. There may be local variations that you need to take account of, in some areas for instance practices nurses are more plentiful and take on a large range of duties. In other areas the district nursing team undertakes most of the discharge care.

Within healthcare there is always some type of waiting involved and referrals are no exception. A referral made in hospital may require follow-up in the community. In the case of a patient needing podiatry (chiropody) care, the referral would be sent out to the community if the patient has been discharged from hospital before being assessed.

How do I refer patients to the community services?

Hospitals will have a list of GP surgeries to be contacted for services such as district nurses, health visitors, practice nurses and other specialist nurses within the community. If your hospital has a discharge coordinator, then they will also have a contact list. If all else fails, look up the patient's GP in the phone directory, call them and seek advice about the services provided by that practice. Recent developments have seen an increase in a number of 'acute' specialties based within the community services. These include services such as 'hospital at home', 'intermediate care', 'first access' and numerous mental health services. It is sometimes difficult to keep on top of these services and most wards will have a 'useful information' book with lists and contact people. Always try phoning and speaking to a named person before commencing any paperwork. Having a named person to contact always gets better results.

Complete the appropriate community referral form. Ensure that it adheres to all the guidelines relating to completion of patient documentation. Document in the patient's records that the referral has been made and the date of referral. Make sure the following details are included:

- Name and address.
- Date of birth.
- GP's name and address.
- Medical history – does the patient have a long-term illness such as diabetes or rheumatoid arthritis?
- Any medication that the patient has been prescribed.
- Clear and concise reason for the referral.
- Date and sign the form.

Helping others to prioritise referrals

If you add URGENT to all community referrals without an explanation, then the person receiving the referral will have no way of prioritising their work. If the referral is urgent, then make that clear on the referral form and add reasons why this is so. An additional telephone call to the person in question will enable you to highlight the urgent needs of this particular patient. That person will also be happy to answer any queries you may have with regard to referrals – just pick up the phone and ask. Do not forget to inform patients of the approximate time interval, e.g. days, weeks or months, before they can expect to be contacted by the referred service.

How do I refer patients to the multidisciplinary team?
Tracey Kemmett and John Fowler

General principles when referring patients

Good communication and early planning are key to all referrals. When you are new to an area try and take some time to meet as many as possible of the other staff involved in the multidisciplinary team. At times the general structure of our work and the busyness of the clinical areas means that staff come onto the ward, carry out clinical duties and then leave. This means that we often do not get the chance to get to know them. So it is vitally important to take time and meet staff; a good professional relationship will help when you are busy.

At first the paperwork and general systems can be a little confusing and not every area has a clear step-by-step process identified. Each service will have a specific referral form that will need to be completed. Find out where these forms are located, what information is required and where they need to be sent once they are completed. Ensure that the referral is recorded in the patient's documentation, including the date, whom the referral has been sent to and your signature and designation. The multidisciplinary team can include physiotherapists, occupational therapists, dietitians, podiatrists, speech therapists, counsellors and many others.

When and why should I refer patients to the multidisciplinary team?

This will depend on the assessed needs of the patient. As a nurse, you will assess, plan and deliver the nursing care required by the patient, but will need to refer the patient to other members of the multidisciplinary team for either advice or specific treatment. It is when the patient requires more than just nursing care that a referral will be needed. If in doubt, have a word with the various allied health professionals and ask their advice. Even busy people will take time to help new staff adjust and fit into a new role. In all cases it is better to make a referral straight away to maximise the recovery of the patient.

If you are new to an area and have a short preceptorship period, then try and take time to spend a couple of hours with all the allied health professionals that input into your area. It is so important to be able to say to your patient what it is like in the physio department, or what happens on an 'OT home visit'. In brief this is an overview:

- *Physiotherapists* concentrate on strength and movement of the body. They can help patients to adapt to certain illnesses or operative procedures. They plan rehabilitation programmes, aiming to enhance patients' recovery. If walking aids are likely to be required following an operation, a referral preoperatively would be appropriate.

- *Occupational therapists* work in conjunction with physiotherapists to enhance a patient's rehabilitation. Their work may involve making support splints to immobilise a joint, assessing the need for dressing aids or aids for everyday activities such as opening a jar or getting in the bath. They may also work with patients, helping them to find ways of conserving their energy and strength, e.g. patients with dyspnoea.
- *Dietitians* assess the nutritional status of patients and plan a diet to ensure that all their nutritional requirements are met. This may include supplements, nasogastric feeding or a weight loss diet. A patient with a poor dietary intake or a patient who has been newly diagnosed with diabetes will require a referral to the dietitian.
- *Podiatrists* specialise in feet and gait analysis, and work in hospitals and the community. If you are not sure of their input, contact the hospital department for advice, or ask one to visit your ward area and run a teaching session about their role. Cutting a patient's toenails can be a nurse's role only when you have been trained how to do this: if not, a referral is required.
- *Speech therapists* would be needed whenever a patient has difficulty in producing words or sounds, e.g. following trauma, maxillary surgery or a stroke, or for swallowing assessment for patients with dysphagia.

How do I refer patients to the multidisciplinary team?

In most wards, regular meetings take place between the nursing staff and members of the multidisciplinary team. Discussions are carried out as to which patients on the ward may require referral or assessment. If these meetings do not occur or if the referral is urgent, follow the referral system identified in the previous section. Once a member of the multidisciplinary team is seeing a patient, he or she will ensure that a referral is carried out if community involvement is required following discharge.

How do I refer patients to specialist nurses?

Each service will have a specific referral form that will need to be completed. Find out where these forms are located, what information is required and where they need to be sent once they are completed. Ensure that the referral is recorded in the patient's documentation, including the date, whom the referral has been sent to and your signature and designation.

Specialist nurses have practical and theoretical knowledge within a specific area of practice. Sometimes this is an area of traditional nursing practice, such as stoma care, or it may be an area more traditionally associated with medical practice, such as pain. The variety and number of specialist nurses in your area will depend on the size of your hospital and the specialties in it. Specialist nurses commonly cover the following areas: asthma, diabetes, tissue viability, infection control, pain, palliative care, sports medicine, rehabilitation, operating departments and specialist outpatient clinics, such as infertility, surgical reconstructions and many more. Make a point of finding out which specialist nurses are available in your area of work.

When, why and how do I refer patients to specialist nurses?

Consult your local guidelines and policies; there may be a strategy written by the specialist nurse regarding what action to take and when to refer. A common system is to have a link nurse on each ward or unit who has a direct link to the specialist lead. The link nurse can then hold regular teaching sessions, enabling the transfer of up-to-date information from the specialist lead to the ward staff or departmental staff. If such a link system operates within your hospital, find out who the link nurses are, how to contact them and their specific role.

To ensure that patients receive the treatment and care they require, as a general rule you should acknowledge your limitations and be aware of where additional experience or expertise lies. If it is beyond your competence and confidence, consult a more experienced nurse initially for advice. Discuss with the link nurse and, if necessary, the nurse specialist. Do not forget that this may be a unit or trust resource and will not necessarily be located on your ward. If a link nurse is not available or is unable to help you, the hospital will have a list of contact numbers to enable you to refer the patient to the specialist nurse. It may be that the medical consultant has advised you to involve the specialist nurse, so you do not have to make that decision.

As with all referrals, always be clear and concise with your information. Ask yourself why you are seeking another's input, document the referral in the patient's records and never be afraid to ask for advice. Do not try to cope if you are not sure what to do – other professionals or specialists are there to help you provide the best care for your patient. Other professionals will not only be happy to answer any questions you have, but will also pass on some valuable knowledge to you in the process.

What are my rights and responsibilities regarding risk management?

Paul Rigby

The assessment and management of risk, partly as a result of clinical governance requirements, now has a much higher profile within clinical practice and is an important part of the nurse's role (Torgesen, 2008). The identification of any potential threats to patient safety and the introduction of measures which aim to eliminate or reduce risk is now part of everyday clinical practice (Bird and Dennis, 2005). *The Code: Standards of Conduct, Performance and Ethics for Nurses and Midwives* (NMC, 2008) outlines clearly the responsibilities that registered nurses have to act to identify to minimise the risk to patients and clients. These are:

- You must act without delay if you believe that you, a colleague or anyone else may be putting someone at risk.
- You must inform someone in authority if you experience problems that prevent you from working within the NMC Code or other nationally agreed standards.
- You must report your concerns in writing if problems in the environment of care are putting people at risk.

Risk assessment and risk management

People often confuse the very different concepts of risk assessment and risk management, and a clear understanding of the differences is a useful starting point for any examination of risk.

- *Risk assessment* involves identifying, through the systematic collection of information, and defining what can go wrong in a situation, and predicting and measuring the likelihood of harm occurring.
- *Risk management* is the measures taken to control risks or to minimise their occurrence.

While it is not possible to eliminate all risks, nurses have a duty to avoid taking unnecessary risks and to protect patients in their care as far as they are able to do so (National Patient Safety Agency, 2007). Doyle (1998) has described a cycle of risk management, which can provide a useful frame of reference when considering the management of risk in clinical practice. (*Figure 5.4*).

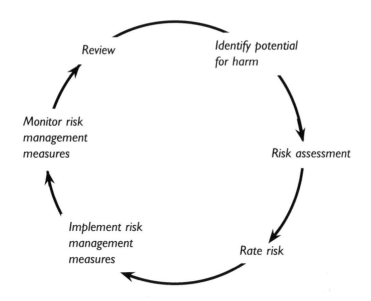

Figure 5.4. Risk management cycle (Doyle, 1998).

Aims of risk assessment and risk management

Raven (1999) has identified four basic aims of risk assessment/ management:

• Protection and safety of the patient/family/community.
• Minimising/reducing risk.
• Minimising litigation risk (personal/organisational).
• Involvement of the patient/carer in the risk assessment/management process.

While there is an increasing number of clinical risk assessment tools available for the nurse to use, it is important to bear in mind certain principles that accompany the process:

• Clinical risk assessment often involves patients and therefore can be an interpersonal process.
• Although clinical risk assessment tools can be very useful, you do need to draw from a wide variety of sources for your information.
• Risk assessments should be grounded in history and based upon empirical evidence.

- You need to focus upon probability rather than certainty.
- Rather than focusing upon at-risk people, you should focus upon at-risk situations (Ryrie, 2000).
- Risk assessment and risk management responsibilities should be shared within the multiprofessional team.

Effective teamworking and decision making are essential components of successful risk management. Risk management is an ongoing process and the opinions of all team members should be sought on a regular basis. Use reflection and your clinical supervision to seek support, share ideas and solve problems.

Clear, objective and accurate record keeping is an important responsibility for all nurses (NMC, 2008). To maintain public confidence it is important that practice is seen to be not only professional and evidence based, but also accountable (Department of Health, 2000c). Even if mistakes are made, it is important that the appropriate lessons are learnt and the necessary changes to practice are made.

As a registered nurse, you have a responsibility to highlight deficiencies in training, communication, teamwork and clinical supervision as well as direct patient care; it is important to bear in mind that all of these factors can affect the process of assessing and managing risk.

What do I need to know about clinical governance?
Flo Brett and Deborah Dowsett

You have possibly heard of clinical governance and consider it yet another jargon term, the latest management talk. You may feel it is 'something meaning nothing' and that it has nothing to do with you. As a newly qualified registered nurse my reaction was similar, but as I gained more experience and began to understand what clinical governance involves and how it can influence patient care, I started to realise that it was going to help me, not hinder me.

What is clinical governance?

Although clinical governance is prominent in modern healthcare, it is often perceived as an abstract concept which has little or nothing to do with day-to-day patient care. This is far from the truth. Clinical governance is about assuring sustainable clinical quality assurance and improvement which can only be achieved by the determined and continuous efforts of clinical and non-clinical staff who have the appropriate support of their organisation to deliver best practice (Sale, 2005).

Clinical governance is an umbrella term used to describe the systematic approach to managing quality control and to assuring the quality of patient care. For me clinical governance can be described as system that 'governs' clinical quality. It is seen as the system designed to improve patient care. The Government White Paper (Department of Health, 1998) emphasised the importance of involving patients and the public not only in gathering their views about care and the services they receive but also through their contribution to NHS policy and planning decisions. So the overall purpose of clinical governance is to ensure that the patient receives the best quality of care that the NHS can provide.

Will it affect my practice and should I know more about it?

As I mentioned earlier, clinical governance is an umbrella term. This implies that it is made up of a number of systems and processes within the organisation for monitoring and improving services. Some of the key components are:

- Patient and public involvement.
- Risk management.
- Clinical audit.
- Clinical effectiveness.

- Staff and staff management.
- Education and training and continuous professional development.
- The use of information technology to support clinical governance and consequently healthcare delivery.

(Nicholls et al, 2000; Starey, 2001)

For this reason it is implicit in your practice as a registered nurse and your day-to-day care. For example, what do you do if you feel a patient is unsafe? When do you provide a clinical incident report? What further education and training do you require to fulfil your role competently and safely? How do you go about organising this? What do you do if a patient makes a complaint? All of these require the appropriate clinical governance systems and processes to be in place to ensure good quality care can be achieved.

Who is responsible for the implementation of clinical governance?

Clinical governance is the responsibility of all staff, clinical and non-clinical, who work together for the benefit of the patient within the healthcare organisation to make it happen. There are specific leads for the clinical governance agenda within most healthcare organisations but implementation of the agenda is everyone's responsibility.

Where did clinical governance come from?

Clinical governance was first introduced into the NHS in 1997 as a comprehensive framework to improve the quality of care for patients. The driving forces behind the clinical governance agenda can be found in the following documents:

- *The New NHS: Modern, Dependable* (Department of Health, 1997). This document sets out a modernisation programme to deliver more consistent, higher quality care.
- *A First Class Service: Quality in the New NHS* (Department of Health, 1998).

These documents detail a framework for quality improvement outlining clear lines of responsibility and accountability for the overall quality of clinical care.

The origins of clinical governance date back to the aftermath of some highly published failures in the NHS in the 1990s which all caused widespread public and political concern and heightened the awareness of the potential for harm (Braine, 2006). These cases also engendered a period of reflection and analysis among health professionals and clinical managers and fostered growing interest in the way health services were managed and delivered. Clinical governance is therefore seen as the framework that is designed to help doctors, nurses and other health professionals to improve clinical standards within the NHS and through which 'organisations are accountable for continuously improving the quality of their services and safeguarding high standards of care by creating an environment in which excellence in clinical care can flourish' (NHS Executive, 1999).

Why do I need to know about clinical governance?

Clinical governance establishes that assuring the quality of patient care is at the centre of the NHS and its key components are familiar to you as a nurse as these concepts also appear in the NMC Code of Professional Conduct (2008). Through the systems and processes that are intrinsic to clinical governance it can also help you to:

- Deliver safe, up-to-date practice.
- Create a patient-centred culture, where patients are informed about their care.
- Minimise clinical errors and prevent these from occurring whenever possible.
- Treat patients courteously and involve them in decisions.
- Ensure patient services are continuously improved.
- Help healthcare professionals to ensure that they keep up to date in their practice.

Important aspects of clinical governance

Clinical governance is your responsibility and not to be ignored. To implement clinical governance, as a staff nurse you will need to collaborate with your colleagues to work to promote and support:

- A learning environment.
- An open culture where staff share ideas and experiences to enhance patient care within the trust and with others outside the organisation.
- Team working where multidisciplinary teams work effectively together.
- Active involvement of patients and carers to inform improvements in our service.

What can I do within my role to help make clinical governance work?

- Have an open mind about new ways of doing things.
- Practice professional self-regulation and ensure you and your colleagues adhere to the policies and processes in place to protect patients and ensure you and your colleagues are fit for practice.
- Apply evidence-based standards to your everyday practice – ask why you do things the way you do and what is the evidence to support your decisions.
- Maintain your own professional development.
- Take part in clinical audit within your area.
- Think about ways to improve how you do things, and share ideas with colleagues.
- Talk to your manager if you are concerned that standards or practices could be improved and think of ways that you could share in this.

Clinical governance should be viewed as an opportunity to improve patient care. It affects all staff regardless of their position within their healthcare organisation. Every nurse has a role within clinical governance which can be realised through maintaining competence to practise safely and effectively, by managing risk, working collaboratively and, perhaps more importantly, being receptive to change and reflective in your approach to care delivery.

References

Alderson P (1993) *Children's Consent to Surgery*. Open University Press, Buckingham

Andrews M (1996) Using reflection to develop clinical expertise. *British Journal of Nursing* **5**(8): 508–13

Andrews M, Chilton F (2000) Student and mentor perceptions of mentoring effectiveness. *Nurse Education Today* **20**(7): 555–62

Benner P (1984) *From Novice to Expert: Excellence and Power in Clinical Nursing Practice*. Addison-Wesley Publishing Company, California

Bowling A (1997) *Research Methods in Health*. Open University Press, Milton Keynes

Braine ME (2006) Clinical Governance: Applying theory to practice. *Nursing Standard* **20**: 26–65

Cahill H (1996) A qualitative analysis of student nurses' experiences of mentorship. *Journal of Advanced Nursing* 24(4): 791–9

Department of Health (1997) *The New NHS: Modern, Dependable*. Cm 3807. The Stationery Office, London

Department of Health (1998) *A First Class Service: Quality in the new NHS*. The Stationery Office, London

Department of Health (2000a) *Patient Group Directions (England only)*. HSC2000/026. Health & Safety Commission, London

Department of Health (2000b) *A Health Service of All the Talents: Developing the NHS workforce*. Consultation document on the review of workforce planning. NHS Executive, Leeds

Department of Health (2000c) *An Organisation with a Memory: Report of an expert group on learning from adverse events in the NHS*. The Stationery Office, London

Department of Health (2004) *Standards for Better Health*. http://www. Department of Health.gov.uk/en/Publicationsandstatistics/Publications/ PublicationsPolicyAndGuidance/Department of Health_4

Doyle M (1998) Clinical risk assessment for mental health nurses. *Nursing Times* **94**(17): 47–9

Earnshaw GJ (1995) Mentorship: The students' views. *Nurse Education Today* **11**: 225–9

English National Board for Nursing, Midwifery and Health Visiting (2001) *Placements in Focus: Guidance for eduction in practice for health care professions*. EMB, London

Fowler J (Ed) (1999) *The Handbook of Clinical Supervision*. Quay Books, Dinton, Wiltshire

Gibbs G (1988) *Learning by Doing: A guide to teaching and learning methods*. Further Education Unit, Oxford Brookes University, Oxford

Glen S, Cox H (2006) E-learning in Nursing: The context. In: Glen S, Moule P (eds) *E-Learning in Nursing*. Palgrave Macmillan, Basingstoke

Glen S, Parker P (2003) *Supporting Learning in Practice – A Guide for Practitioners*. Palgrave Macmillan, London

Gray MA, Smith LN (2000) The qualities of an effective mentor from the student nurse's perspective: Findings from a longitudinal qualitative study. *Journal of Advanced Nursing* **32**(6): 1542–9

Griffith R, Tengnah C (2008) *Law and Professional Issues in Nursing*. Learning Matters Limited, Exeter

Hindle T (1998) *Reducing Stress*. Dorling Kindersley, London

Hulatt I (1995) A sad reflection. *Nursing Standard* **9**(20): 22–3

Jarvis P (1992) Reflective practice and nursing. *Nurse Education Today* **12**(3): 174–81

Jarvis P, Gibson S (Eds) (1997) *The Teacher Practitioner and Mentor in Nursing, Midwifery and Health Visiting and the Social Services* (2nd edn). Stanley Thornes, Cheltenham

Johns C (2000) *Becoming a Reflective Practitioner*. Blackwell Science, London

Knowles M (1973) *The Adult Learner: A neglected species*. Gulf Publishing Company, Houston, Texas

Knowles M (1980) *The Modern Practice of Adult Education: From Pedagogy to Andragogy*. Follett, Chicago, Illinois

Lloyd Jones M, Walters S, Akehurst R (2001) The implications of contact with the mentor for preregistration nursing and midwifery students. *Journal of Advanced Nursing* **35**(2): 151–60

Locasto LW, Kochanek D (1989) Reality Shock in the Nurse Educator. *Journal of Nursing Education* **28**(2): 79–81

Martin V (2000) Managing your time. Part 3. *Nursing Times* **96**(18): 42

Maslow AH (1943) A theory of human motivation. *Psychology Review* **50**: 370–96

McSherry R, Kell J, Pearce P (2002) Clinical supervision and clinical governance. *Nursing Times* **98**(23): 30–2

Morton-Cooper A, Palmer A (1993) *Mentoring, Preceptorship and Clinical Supervision: A guide to professional roles in clinical practice* (2nd edn). Blackwell Science, Oxford

National Patient Safety Agency (2007) *Healthcare Risk Made Easy*. NHS NPSA, London

Neary M, Phillips R, Davies B (1994) *The Practitioner Teacher: A study in the introduction of mentors in pre-registration Nurse Education Programme in Wales*. School of Education, University of Wales, Cardiff

Newman M, Roberts T (2002) Critical appraisal 2: Can the evidence be applied in your context? In: Craig JV, Smyth RL (eds) *The Evidence-Based Practice Manual for Nurses*. Churchill Livingstone, Edinburgh

NHS Executive (1999) *Clinical Governance Quality in the New NHS. Health Service Circular HSC 1999/065*. The Stationary Office, London.

Nicholls S, Cullen R, O'Neill S, Halligan A (2000) Clinical Governance: Its origins and its foundations. *Clinical Performance and Quality in Health Care* **8**(3): 172–8

Nursing and Midwifery Council (2002) *Supporting Nurses and Midwives Through*

Lifelong Learning. NMC, London

Nursing and Midwifery Council (2004) *The PREP Handbook*. Nursing and Midwifery Council, London

Nursing and Midwifery Council (2008) *Standards to Support Learning and Assessment in Practice: Nursing and Midwifery Council Standards for Mentors, Practice Teachers and Teachers*. Nursing and Midwifery Council, London.

Polit D, Hungler B (1995) *Nursing Research: Principles and Methods*. Lippincott, Philadelphia

Raven J (1999) Managing the unmanageable: Risk assessment and risk management in contemporary professional practice. *Journal of Nursing Management* **7**(4): 201–6

Ryrie I (2000) Assessing risk. In: Gamble C, Brennan G (eds). *Working with Serious Mental Illness: A manual for clinical practice*. Baillière Tindall/RCN, London

Sale D (2005) *Understanding Clinical Governance and Quality Assurance – Making it Happen*. Palgrave Macmillan, Basingstoke

Shepperd S, Doll H, Jenkinson C (1997) Randomized controlled trials. Cited in Scott C (1999) A description of the roles, activities and skills of clinical nurse specialists in the United States. *Clinical Nurse Specialist* **13**(4): 183–90

Snowball R (1999) Finding the evidence: An information skills approach. In: Dawes M, Davies P, Gray A, Mant J et al (eds) *Evidence Based Practice: A primer for healthcare professionals*. Churchill Livingstone, Edinburgh

Spouse J (1996) The effective mentor: A model for student-centred learning. *Nursing Times* **92**(13): 32–5

Starey N (2001) What is Clinical Governance? *Evidence Based Medicine* 1(12): 1–8

Thompson C, Learmouth M (2002) How can we develop an evidence-based culture? In: Craig JV, Smyth RL (eds) T*he Evidence-Based Practice Manual for Nurses*. Churchill Livingstone, Edinburgh

Torgesen I (2008) Risk management. *Nursing Times* **104**(17): 12–13

United Kingdom Central Council for Nursing, Midwifery and Health Visiting (1994) *The Council's Standards for Education and Practice following Registration: Programmes leading to the Qualification of Specialist Practitioner.* UKCC, London

Wheeler J (2001) Staff development through appraisal. *Nursing Times* **97**(39): 34

Notes

Index